The Longest Loss: Alzheimer's Disease and Dementia

Edited by Kenneth J. Doka and Amy S. Tucci

Foreword by Peter V. Rabins

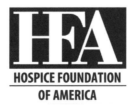

HOSPICE FOUNDATION
OF AMERICA

This book is part of Hospice Foundation of America's *Living with Grief®* series.

This book is part of HFA's *Living with Grief*® series.

Ordering information:

Call Hospice Foundation of America: 800-854-3402

Or write:
Hospice Foundation of America
1710 Rhode Island Avenue, NW #400
Washington, DC 20036

Or visit HFA's Web site:
www.hospicefoundation.org

Managing Editor: Lisa McGahey Veglahn
Editorial Assistance: Spencer Levine
Layout and Design: HBP, Inc.

Publisher's Cataloging-in-Publication
(Provided by Quality Books, Inc.)

    The longest loss : Alzheimer's disease and dementia /
      edited by Kenneth J. Doka and Amy S. Tucci.
      pages cm
      Includes bibliographical references and index.
      LCCN 2014958628
      ISBN 978-1-893349-18-6

      1. Alzheimer's disease.   2. Alzheimer's disease—
    Patients—Care. 3. Caregivers.   4. Bereavement.
    5. Grief.   I. Doka, Kenneth J., editor. II. Tucci, Amy
    S., editor. III. Hospice Foundation of America.

RC523.L66 2015   616.8'31
                         QBI15-600020

Dedication

To Elvira "Vera" Mezzacuella

*In deep appreciation for her help and
secretarial assistance for over 30 years*

KJD

To caregivers of individuals with dementia

AST

Contents

Acknowledgments

We thank our staff of the Hospice Foundation of America: Spencer Levine, Kristen Nanjundaram, Lindsey Currin, and Aziza Jones. They accomplish so much. We appreciate their devotion to our mission at the Hospice Foundation of America.

We also wish to recognize our outstanding managing editor Lisa McGahey Veglahn. Lisa oversees deadlines, keeps authors – and editors – on track, and carefully reviews all aspects of production.

Naturally, we also need to thank the authors who respond to our tight deadlines. We are extremely fortunate that we are able to maintain an "A" list of authors. This year is no exception. We especially appreciated those who shared their personal stories.

Both editors thank their families and friends for their patience as we struggle to publish a book on such a tight timetable. Both editors benefit from the respite and grounding these family and friends offer.

As always, we wish to thank the Hospice Foundation of America's Board of Directors and all the organizations and individuals that support our efforts.

Foreword

Peter V. Rabins

In the space of 40 years, what was once termed "senility" is now widely recognized and feared as resulting from a group of diseases clustered under the term "dementia." While the medicalization of life has drawbacks, the benefits of recognizing that the development of cognitive impairment in adulthood is the result of a number of distinct diseases has resulted in many benefits to those with these diseases and those who care for them. Chief among them is the recognition that these disorders of the brain, including Alzheimer's disease, which accounts for about two-thirds of cases, are progressive and require a wide range of services along their course.

While each of more than 80 diseases that cause dementia differs in many ways, those that are neurodegenerative, that is, cause the progressive death of central nervous system cells, ultimately end in death. Indeed, a recent Centers for Disease Control and Prevention (CDC) report found that death rates from cardiovascular disease and cancer have fallen in recent years but have risen for dementia.

One of the unique characteristics of the diseases that cause dementia is that some are associated with a loss of insight at the onset of the illness, but almost all that are progressive are associated with loss of insight when they become severe. This reality has significant impact on caring for those with the disease.

Another unique aspect of the dementias is that they often lead to changes in personality and behavior. In Alzheimer's disease, for example, my colleague Martin Steinberg has shown that 60% of individuals with dementia are experiencing one or more behavioral or neuropsychiatric symptoms at any one time and that 90% experience at least one such symptom sometime in the course of the disease.

A third unique aspect of the dementias is that a whole system of facility-based care has developed to care for the one-third of individuals with dementia whose illness can no longer be taken care of at home. Today, more than 3 million Americans live in nursing homes or assisted living facilities, approximately 70% of whom have dementia.

On the other hand, the dementias are similar to other diseases that change the course of life and lead to death. All such illnesses are associated with a grieving process in both the person with dementia and those who love and care for them. It is this that is the focus of this book.

The Longest Loss: Alzheimer's Disease and Dementia brings together an impressive group of experts who provide important information on both the similarities with other life situations and the unique aspects of the grieving process experienced by those who have dementia and those who are caring for them. By emphasizing that the experience of grief varies as the disease progresses, that the chronicity and decline that are characteristic of the progressive dementias interrupt the adaptation that occurs among those who are dying and in those grieving the death of a loved one, and that the loss of insight characteristic of many dementias raises unique challenges for the person with dementia and for their caregivers, this volume will undoubtedly improve the care provided to a particularly needy and previously underserved group.

Most importantly, by highlighting the fact that grief, that most universal of human experiences, is at the core of dementia care, *The Longest Loss: Alzheimer's Disease and Dementia* will benefit the millions of Americans who are living through, and with, Alzheimer's disease and similar illnesses.

Peter V. Rabins, MD, MPH, has been on the faculty of the Johns Hopkins School of Medicine since 1978. He is the emeritus Richman Family Professor and founding director of the Division of Geriatric Psychiatry and Neuropsychiatry in the Department of Psychiatry and Behavioral Sciences and a member of the Johns Hopkins Berman Bioethics Institute.

Dr. Rabins has spent his career studying psychiatric disorders in the elderly. He was the first to demonstrate elevated mortality in persons with delirium and among the first to identify high rates of neuropsychiatric symptoms in persons with dementia. He is the author or editor of more than 280 peer-reviewed articles and 8 books, including The 36-Hour Day, a Family Guide for People who have Alzheimer Disease, Related Dementias, and Memory Loss *(Johns Hopkins University Press, 2011).*

Introduction

In 2004, Hospice Foundation of America (HFA) focused its *Living With Grief®* program and companion book on Alzheimer's disease. The opening chapter noted that, as Baby Boomers aged, the sheer numbers of individuals with Alzheimer's or other dementias would present a "coming crisis" for hospice. As HFA revisits Alzheimer's disease and other related dementias in 2015, it is clear that this warning was prescient. The 2014 report of the National Hospice and Palliative Care Organization (NHPCO) notes that dementia is now the second most prevalent diagnosis for admission to hospice. The Alzheimer's Association (2014) projects that rate may triple by 2050. The crisis has come.

As the hospice model was originally developed for persons with cancer, the increasing admission of individuals with dementia offers both challenges and opportunities for hospice and palliative care. The challenges are many. Pain management, for example, is far more difficult when patients have dementia. Subtle and not-so-subtle patient cues, as well as caregiver reports, may be required to assess pain.

There is another challenge as well. While Alzheimer's and other forms of dementia are assigned medical stages that mark the progression of the disease, prognosis is still difficult to predict. Even in the last stages of the disease, when patients are expected to die within six months, impairment is significant, and there are concomitant medical conditions, the quality of caregiving and other factors can make such predictions quickly moot.

Yet hospice and palliative care programs have much to offer to persons with dementia and their families. Hospices generally offer home-based care, and hospice caregivers and volunteers are sensitive to the needs of caregivers and their families. They may provide respite care and even offer care continuity if a patient is transferred to a nursing home. Hospice and palliative care professionals are experts in pain management, even with the challenges posed by dementia.

Most importantly, they offer expertise in understanding grief, an aspect of care central to the hospice mission. Grief is a constant companion in dementia, whether it is experienced by the patient or the family. The concept of *anticipatory grief* or *anticipatory mourning* is critical. Therese Rando (2000) redefined anticipatory mourning as grief generated by losses experienced *within* the illness, rather than simply grief generated by an anticipation of future death.

In the early stages of Alzheimer's disease and other dementias, this kind of grief is experienced by the patient as well as the family. Author Thaddeus Rauschi (2004) noted the first time he began to experience cognitive declines, often in seemingly unimportant events such as getting into small fender benders or entering the wrong restroom. His wife commented on "his delayed thinking." After his diagnosis of early stage Alzheimer's, he was able to acknowledge his grief over the many losses he experienced, such as the inability to engage in small talk or participate in community activities as he once did. Rauschi's work, written when he was in the early stages of dementia, reflects the fear of someone who knows he is beginning a frightful decline. Grief is now a companion to him and his family.

Later in the illness, losses compound, generated by both the deterioration of the patient and the losses inherently associated with caregiving. These losses are shared throughout the intimate network but especially by family members most engaged in care. Individuals surrender their own independence to the demands of caregiving. They mourn the loss of the person they once knew even as they care for this stranger now in their midst. Their assumptions of the world may be challenged as well; this was neither what they expected nor wanted. While the person with dementia may not be able to fully understand the losses experienced, he or she often has a sense of *wrongbeing*, a sense that pieces of their personal puzzle seem to be missing.

This is perhaps where hospices and palliative care programs can play a vital role. Hospices often receive patients with dementia so late in the disease that their ability to offer a comprehensive range of support and services is severely constrained. Some hospices have developed innovative partnerships with local chapters of the Alzheimer's Association and other groups for patients and families dealing with dementia. Hospices and palliative care organizations have proven expertise in pain management and supporting families through end-of-life decision making and grief. Dementia-related organizations can profit from this expertise, and hospices can connect in positive ways with families earlier in the disease process.

We hope our program and this book will help. *The Longest Loss: Alzheimer's Disease and Dementia* focuses on the experience of loss within dementia, alternating personal stories and narratives of the disease with chapters authored by some of the leading authorities on grief and dementia.

Nancy Pearce begins the book by addressing a critical question: Do persons with dementia experience grief? Pearce affirms they do. Wisely and sensitively, she reminds us that emotions are distinct from cognition and connections, especially historic connections, generate grief, or at least a sense of loss, when they are missed. Pearce then offers strategies for helping to support persons with dementia as they grieve.

Elizabeth Uppman's narrative of her grandmother's dementia reminds us of the ongoing grief that family members experience as they cope with the loss of someone they love. Doka (2002) notes that, in *psychosocial loss*, we experience the loss of the persona of someone we loved. The person remains alive but the essence of the person we once knew and loved is now gone. Dementia is a classic example of such a loss. Yet Uppman adds a poignant reminder. Every once in a while, we still—even deep in the disease—catch a glimpse of the person we now grieve.

Katherine Supiano's chapter focuses on the grief that dementia caregivers experience both within and after the caregiving experience. The losses experienced in caregiving are profound. One grieves the diminished abilities and the increasing loss of freedom generated when caring for a person with dementia. There is a loss of an assumptive world. We likely never expected such a role when we first said our vows; there was nothing about changing diapers. Nor as children did we ever expect to have our roles with our parents so dramatically reversed. Yet after the death there are other losses, as we mourn the death while simultaneously trying to rebuild a life placed on hold, often even for decades.

Charles and Donna Corr's chapter makes two significant contributions to the discussion. They recount the multigenerational nature of the disease; dementia often does run in families. The Corrs relate their own experiences in caregiving as dementia impacts their lives directly. This very personal perspective reminds us how caregiving can be so readily incorporated into life as a couple. The essay reinforces an important aspect of caregiver burden; the degree of burden depends less on what one has to do and more on what the relationship has been. In the supportive relationship that Charles and Donna have, the burden is much diminished.

Jennifer Elison and Chris McGonigle draw from the extensive work that provided the basis of their groundbreaking book, *Liberating Losses* (2003). Their chapter reminds us that grief is a reaction to loss, and that these reactions can vary. One significant and often overlooked response, especially after the strains of caregiving in dementia, can be *relief*. Here the relief can be *altruistic*, based on the realization that the person who died is no longer suffering. It can be *dual relief*, a feeling that the deceased individual's suffering, and ours, is ended. A final type is *relationship relief*, often found when a relationship has been highly difficult or abusive. Elison and McGonigle's chapter reinforces the varied nature of the grief experience while reminding counselors to probe for such reactions as they may be disenfranchised by the larger society.

Cris Abrams's account of her mother's journey with dementia brings many important reminders. Caring for someone with dementia can be both rewarding and stressful. That stress can create additional sources of grief, such as family rifts. Abrams also reaffirms that, as the disease progresses, care plans may continue to change, generating additional conflict and exacerbating stress. Abrams makes one other subtle but critical point. We often have expectations of how we expect persons with dementia to react to our care—expectations that rarely are fulfilled.

Kenneth Doka concludes the book with a chapter that summarizes the experience of grief throughout dementia. While Doka's chapter reviews the grief experienced both by persons with Alzheimer's disease or other dementias as well as their families and caregivers, he sensitizes us to the grief that might be experienced by professional caregivers. A paradox exists that can generate conflict and misunderstanding between family and professional caregivers. Family caregivers are likely to be grieving the loss of the person prior to the onset of dementia, while professional caregivers are mourning the person they knew, the person impacted and changed by dementia.

These chapters and personal stories reiterate the critical thesis of this book. Grief begins at the very onset of illness and continues well after the death; the grief journey of Alzheimer's disease and dementia is indeed the longest loss.

REFERENCES

Alzheimer's Association. (2014). Facts and figures. Retrieved from http://www.alz.org/alzheimers_disease_facts_and_figures. asp#prevalence.

Doka, K. J. (Ed.) (2002). *Disenfranchised grief: New directions, challenges and strategies for practice.* Champaign, IL: Research Press.

Kapo, J., & Karlawish, J. (2004). Ethical challenges for end-of-life care for dementia patients. In K. J. Doka (Ed.), *Living with grief: Alzheimer's disease* (pp. 255-267). Washington, DC: Hospice Foundation of America.

Elison, J., & McGonigle, C. (2003). *Liberating losses: When death brings relief.* Cambridge, MA: Perseus Books.

National Hospice and Palliative Care Organization. (2014). *NHPCO's facts and figures: Hospice care in America.* Alexandria, VA: NHPCO.

Rando, T. A. (2000). *Clinical dimensions of anticipatory mourning: Theory and practice in working with the dying, their loved ones, and their caregivers.* Champaign, IL: Research Press.

Rauschi, T. (2004). Something was not right. In K. J. Doka (Ed.), *Living with grief: Alzheimer's disease* (pp. 99-110). Washington, DC: Hospice Foundation of America.

CHAPTER 1

Do People with Dementia Experience Grief?

Nancy Pearce

Miss Sophia's 87 years of life were "filled with hardships and sadness, not the least of which flared with the news of Alzheimer's disease 13 years ago," according to Pamela, the niece who helped Miss Sophia stay in her home for most of those years. "It was actually a blessing when Aunt Sophia finally forgot that she forgot." Eventually, her aunt's needs were too extreme for homecare. By the time Miss Sophia came to the skilled care facility where I worked as a social worker, she needed total care from a team of professionals. She was no longer verbal and did not appear to interact with or even recognize her twin sister and dearest companion.

Miss Sophia's first year at the facility went very smoothly. Each day she sat quietly in her wheelchair with hands gently folded on her lap. She appeared to be quite content and smiled at the simplest of things—a colorful picture on the wall, the flavorful spoonful of pureed food, or the sound of a hymn at Sunday services.

One Tuesday evening, however, Miss Sophia's personality dramatically shifted. For the next four days, Miss Sophia rocked back and forth, furrowed her brow, vacillated between sighs and rapid breathing, had difficulty sleeping, resisted food and water, and had long periods of crying. Although staff could calm these behaviors with hugs or by holding her hands, Miss Sophia would revert to her signs of distress soon after they had left. Although we attempted to contact Pamela to talk about what other interventions might be effective, we were unable to reach her.

Four days later, at her usual time, Pamela came to the facility to visit her aunt. We learned that we could not reach Pamela for the past several days because her mother, Miss Sophia's twin sister, had suddenly died that past Tuesday evening. We spent a significant amount of time talking with Pamela, providing our condolences and support before discussing her aunt's condition.

Even with profound cognitive loss and the apparent inability to remember a significant person in her life, Aunt Sophia still had a sense that something was amiss. The person with dementia has very strong antennae and can sense even slight changes in others and the environment. She may sense the inconsistency of presence or feel the change on levels we may not at all understand, such as was possible with Miss Sophia.

Even persons with advanced dementia have the ability to experience grief. If observant, clinicians and other caregivers can see evidence of grief reactions. Even if we only hold the possibility of grief reactions in persons in the later stages of dementia, we as healthcare professionals need to figure out ways to be supportive. Being helpful requires us to stretch our traditional cognitive approaches to the therapeutic process and find ways to enter the person's world in order to walk with him or her through the grief experience. This task begins with heightening our observations while letting go of our opinions, expectations, and assumptions about expressions and processing of grief.

VARIED GRIEF RESPONSES AFTER THE DEATH OF A LOVED ONE

The person with dementia is, first and foremost, a person, with the potential for a full range of emotions that are part of a normal human reaction to the loss of a loved one. Even with advanced dementia, the loss of cognition does not mean loss of the ability to feel and express emotions, so the potential to experience grief remains. We may see evidence of the person's reactions that we commonly associate with grieving, such as sadness, anger, agitation, anxiety, guilt, and other emotions. As the progression of dementia robs her of the words and cognitive abilities to describe and make sense of these feelings and their association with loss, we who offer support must move beyond our normal assumptions with grieving to look for nonverbal cues, such as changes in restlessness, searching or fidgety behaviors, shallow breathing or sighing, changes in skin color and moisture, increased heart rate or respirations, increased sensitivity to noise, changes in sleep and/or appetite, social withdrawal, or increased confusion. This list is as extensive as our ability to pay attention to the smallest detail. Any of these changes may be indications that the person is experiencing a grief reaction.

A person with dementia is like anyone else who is mourning in that her expressions of grief can shift from one moment to the next. Her grief may be affected by the frequency of contact with the deceased and the closeness of their relationship, the degree of cognitive loss, the ability to express her loss to others, even the timeframe in which she believes she is living. (For example, a grief response to the loss of a spouse could potentially be much different if the person with dementia sees herself as a young child.)

We know that her ability to clearly articulate her reactions is dramatically compromised by the progression of the disease, but we cannot assume that these reactions do not occur. She might be dealing with the emotional content of events in a way that is different from what we would normally perceive to be a traditional therapeutic process of grieving. We also may never really know fully how her processing plays out. However her reactions may be manifested, a significant part of our ability to be supportive is that we allow for these emotions to be expressed and that we empathically and compassionately connect. Some basic approaches that appear to be more effective in making connections with a person who has dementia can be extremely useful.

HEARING AND HONORING CONNECTIONS

Working and being with persons who have dementia continues to teach me that my function is less about figuring out specific actions I can take to help, as much as understanding the qualities in my approach. It is not about what I do or do not say; it is not about someone getting anything from me, or my doing to or doing for someone else. As Miller (1997, p. 47) writes, "…it is about being in the flow of human connection rather than out of it." Within this relationship, the healing occurs.

My observations tell me that when a person with dementia is in a connected state with others, she has a greater potential for increased clarity, a greater potential for insights or "aha!" moments, and a greater potential for connecting to levels of self and others—the energy field that some call the "other side" or "heaven."

The list of "dos" and "don'ts" is not as important as the way we enter the moment with the person who has dementia. When we relax our hold on how we see ourselves, release our need to know or to be right about the specifics, and dare to stretch outside our standard operating mode, we become free to explore how the person is currently experiencing her world. Being with her in her experience is how the connection and healing process will evolve.

Anyone can do this; it simply takes time, patience, and a willingness to be open. There are no "shoulds" or "have-tos," just two basic concepts to follow.

Getting out of the way

A person with dementia senses and reacts to whatever tensions, distractions, apathy, judgments, or opinions we may be presenting in any given moment, even though we think we are disguising them. As the disease progresses, she will become less able to find words or link concepts that help make sense of why the interaction either does or does not feel right. But her reaction, even when totally nonverbal, will reflect our own attitudes. Truly notice, listen, and pay attention in the moment. Allow the person with dementia to be your guide and teach you how to proceed.

One way to begin is to take a moment to breathe deeply and try to allow past and future concerns or worries to flow out of your body. As you breathe, bring your attention to various parts of your body to "take a reading." Where you read tension, try allowing it to slip away with the exhaling of your breath. Bring your full attention to this process, allowing all other thoughts to slip away as you breathe out. Slow down. Become fully aware of yourself in the moment (Pearce, 2011).

Open stance

Once you let go of whatever could be getting in the way, it is important to bring yourself to an open place. By "open," I am referring to feeling respect, strong admiration, warm attachment, compassion, and kindness toward the person you are about to meet. The open place is the essential mortar in the bridge between any caregiver and the person with dementia.

When your attention, intention, and focus are on holding the person with dementia in tender and positive regard, you will exude real warmth. This warmth creates an open, spacious, and receptive likelihood for connection. Without the warmth that you bring to the moment, creating an authentic relationship with the person who has dementia will be a challenge.

As you approach the person with dementia while thinking about what you like and admire about him or her, you enter the moment in an open and positive state. He or she sees and hears this in your body stance, your voice, your facial expressions, and your words, possibly without you even being aware of your physical and vocal qualities. You become calm and as gently relaxed as a close friend because you are holding positive feelings in your heart. All of these manifestations of your shift toward openness will be effective in interacting with persons who have dementia. Yet it appears that the impact of our open, calming presence may go beyond these things we can immediately identify.

Exciting research has been done at the Institute of HeartMath, the results from which are published in *The HeartMath Solution* (1999) and *Transforming Stress* (2005). Their research shows that positive emotions such as compassion, love, and joy produce smooth or more ordered heart rhythm patterns which, in turn, are associated with physical, mental, and emotional health. Some of the research shows how heart rhythms, both smooth and irregular, produce electromagnetic signals that have been measured beyond the body up to 10 feet away. The electromagnetic signals that emit from the rhythms of a person's heart have also been measured in the brain waves of other persons nearby. These studies indicate that we are literally making waves as we feel our emotions and those waves affect the heart rhythms and brain waves of persons around us. This energetic nonverbal communication via heart rhythms produces an immediate and deep understanding and connection between human beings.

When we enter each moment with positive emotions and their associated smooth heart rhythms, we help the person with dementia to do the same. Smooth heart rhythms give each of us a greater potential for adapting to stressful events, for improving overall health and well-being, and for improving communication and connection. As you remain open to connecting with the person, the intention is to find the essential emotion within his or her story and respond in relation to his or her truth about the world, in that moment, on that day. Once you identify his or her emotion, find ways to empathize with that feeling. To empathize successfully, focus on the emotion and not merely on the facts as presented. Minimize your tendency to analyze and interpret details; it is simply inappropriate to do so, as is debate or disagreement with his or her truth. To dig too deeply into, or to challenge the facts or details of, what is being said keeps both of you in separate versions of reality and locks out any hope of connection. The person with dementia believes the reasons for his or her feelings and that need for self-expression is valid. That is enough.

Allowing yourself to temporarily identify with the experience of the person with dementia and see it from his or her perspective is an essential way into connection; even in a small way, this process helps bridge the gap that separates us. Reflecting your identification with the person with dementia signals that he or she was heard and is not alone.

"Being with" someone who has dementia is not about merely staying in her presence, being nice, and providing a forum for talking or just hanging out (not that there's anything wrong with that). Being with this person is your opportunity to remain outwardly and inwardly silent as an attentive presence, so that you can hear and enter the truth of his or her experience, with or without its verbal and nonverbal expressions. In open silence, you can identify and listen to the emotional truth that the person with dementia needs to express. By being available, you get the extraordinary chance to really see, accept, and empathize without judgment, and to validate the emotions and the person. It is this quality of the griever-listener relationship that will promote the greatest healing.

How Should the Death of a Loved One Be Communicated?

When dementia enters the equation, we appear to become frozen with concerns and over-complications rather than going back to essential concepts. We tend to assume that traditional cognitive models of grief work are inappropriate when supporting a person whose cognition shifts from one moment to the next and whose ability to retain insights does not appear to exist. Two common aspects of these models can be very helpful in helping a person who has dementia cope with grief. These models posit that there will be some emotional responses to the loss, such as shock, confusion, anxiety, or guilt, that will be expressed verbally and nonverbally; yet the griever has the potential to move through this process to incorporate the loss in his or her life. The process of grieving is unique and individual; each person grieves in his or her own way and time. The person with dementia may not remember the reality of the loss from moment to moment, yet may be able to work through the emotions with a compassionate listener and adjust to the loss over time.

This brings us back to Miss Sophia. Pamela's primary question was whether she should tell Miss Sophia about her twin sister's death, worrying that, "she has enough to deal with without all of this!" The general consensus among professionals is that a person with dementia needs to be told at least once about the death of a person who was a part of everyday life or with whom he or she had a significant relationship. Persons with dementia are generally very sensitive, and highly responsive, to the emotional states of those around them. If other family members are grieving, the person with dementia may perceive those emotions and become distressed, without being able to cognitively process why. She may be grieving without understanding what it is about, as many of us believed was true with Miss Sophia.

I would much rather err on the side of assuming that the person with dementia, even in the later stages of the illness, can understand and enter the process of grieving the loss. Many times, the person with dementia will enter into a particular moment of clarity and will clearly express an understanding of the situation. She may notice the deceased is no longer visiting; something has changed, or has become lost or unfamiliar in her routine. The person with dementia may sense this at some other level beyond the rational, such as was possible with Miss Sophia. Affording the person with dementia the opportunity to share feelings of grief is important.

Pamela requested a team meeting to create a plan to tell Miss Sophia about her sister's death. This team consisted of staff members who were most acquainted with Miss Sophia: the nurse, physician, social worker, spiritual counselor, therapeutic activities director, food service worker, a particular volunteer, and her favorite nursing assistant. Everyone on the team agreed that Miss Sophia needed to be told about her sister's death, even though she seemed to already know on some inexplicable level. Her behaviors could be interpreted as grieving reactions and they were so perfectly timed with her sister's death. We agreed it was important to explore ideas as to what would be the most effective, compassionate approach in informing and supporting Miss Sophia.

Our goal was to come up with an individualized care plan that would maximize Miss Sophia's strengths to support her in her grieving. Since she was a very private person who preferred one-on-one connections, we agreed that it would be best to have just one person, someone well-known to her, give her the news. Although Pamela was the logical choice, we assured her that if her own grief was too overwhelming, we could suggest another family member, friend, or team member to be of assistance. Pamela was very clear that she was in a "good place" and that it could be a potentially bonding experience with her aunt. She only felt insecure about how to proceed and what to say.

We talked with Pamela about how a simple, honest, compassionate approach is best, using short sentences and clear words like "died" rather than euphemisms such as "crossed over" or "passed on." We encouraged her to answer Miss Sophia's questions, if any arose, as honestly as possible. For example, explaining the deceased person's absence by stating that he or she is "away and will come another day" can backfire. The deceased's return may be the only piece of information the listener retains and can increase agitation and worry when that person does not come.

We assured Pamela that she should provide support if Miss Sophia expressed or showed signs of emotion, but to be prepared that she might not have any reaction at all; she may not seem to be distressed in the moment she is told about the death. We also reminded Pamela that Miss Sophia may never react or respond to the information, or that she may bring it up repetitively over time. The goal would not be to force her into a certain reality but to find ways to accompany her wherever she is.

The focus shifted to creating a list of Miss Sophia's strongest coping tools that we felt could help support her in times of grieving or stress: her love of Mozart piano concertos, a certain stuffed animal, arranging playing cards in order, or simply holding hands. All of these things had helped Miss Sophia feel more at peace and be more engaged in the past. We agreed to keep the team updated as other strengths emerged.

In most cases, informing the person with dementia as soon as possible, taking into account his or her strengths and even the best time of day for them, is the best approach. With Miss Sophia, we all felt that the conversation needed to happen as soon as possible. Most of the team sensed that Miss Sophia was grieving and needed active support, and we were concerned that Miss Sophia would pick up on Pamela's or a team member's sadness or sense that something was not the same.

In reference to the setting that would best meet Miss Sophia's needs, we all agreed that the most supportive environment would be private, quiet, and free from distractions. Possible considerations to maximize a positive dialogue with persons with dementia, especially those who are elderly, are sound (possibly playing calming music in the background); lighting (particularly if there are visual deficits); visual beauty (flowers or other favorite objects); and touch.

We also discussed the importance of having staff members stay close to Miss Sophia after the discussion to observe for reactions and provide comfort and support. All of the tips we created were added to Miss Sophia's 24-hour plan of care so they would be communicated to all shifts.

Pamela felt prepared but requested that the social worker remain available during the conversation. Pamela took Miss Sophia to the pond outside the facility, a place she knew had always relaxed her, and briefly told Miss Sophia that her sister had died suddenly from a heart attack. They hugged and cried for a period of time and then sat quietly, just holding hands. After about 20 minutes, Pamela began to cry again. Miss Sophia lifted her hand and placed it over Pamela's heart, using a gesture Pamela's mother had used to comfort her when she was young. Pamela knew she was being comforted by Miss Sophia.

This image touches on another reason why it is important to inform the person with dementia of a loved one's death: telling the person may be important for the family caregiver. Family members and the person with dementia have the potential of being with each other during this time in a mutually beneficial, empowering, and supportive way.

We tracked Miss Sophia's behaviors over time to see if the information helped create a shift in her challenging behaviors. Her incidences of being upset were significantly reduced immediately following her meeting with Pamela, going from almost constant to only once a day for most days. These moments were also more easily shifted; each time Miss Sophia showed signs of distress, she was easily consoled when staff would give her a hug and say, "I'm so sorry, Miss Sophia." Each time, she became calm and appeared content for the rest of the day. After several weeks, these episodes no longer occurred.

The team agreed that there was no need to continually bring up the death; instead, they would allow Miss Sophia to take the lead, even nonverbally, through changes in behavior. During the weeks following the meeting, Pamela actively involved Miss Sophia in memorial planning and the burial of the urn. We were surprised at how Miss Sophia was able to be clear about the funeral rituals, religious passages, and music that she wanted at the memorial service. We also felt that these familiarities helped keep her more focused and present during the service. Miss Sophia's favorite picture of her sister was placed up front as a good visual focusing tool. The length of the service was shortened and planned for early in the day to match Miss Sophia's limitations and energy level. We also arranged for a favorite aide to be with her during the service in case she needed to leave. All present actively shared grieving with each other in the form of reminiscing and story-telling. Miss Sophia's synopsis at the end of the service was a gentle and slow "Hmmmm…" with a smile.

When The Questioning Keeps Coming

A straightforward approach worked effectively for Miss Sophia, for which we were all thankful. It is important to note that not all situations go so smoothly; after all, dementia is neither predictable nor logical. One of the most frustrating situations for caregivers is when we have thoughtfully shared the information with a person with dementia that a loved one has died and spent a significant amount of time supporting them through grief reactions and emotions, only to have the person apparently forget the information, efforts, and compassionate focus by bringing up the deceased as if nothing happened. We breathe to try to settle down our own reactions and give perhaps yet another gentle reminder that the person died, but the questioning may continue fresh each new moment or each new day.

Gradually over time (or sometimes very quickly), most of us begin to realize how frustrating this process, and this disease, can be. How many times can we answer the same question, particularly if we have our own grief over the loss, before it begins to wear on our patience? Of course we understand that the person's inability to remember is a result of a disease process. It may be destruction of brain tissue and/or structural changes in the brain, but something has occurred in the brain that has interrupted her ability to interact and remember in predictable ways. Yet this clinical understanding is not always enough to stop us from experiencing a full range of human emotions and reactions when asked repeated questions. What can be done when our usual ways of responding do not appear to work?

The unfortunate reality is that there is no one answer or step to take to deal with the repetitive questioning. People's personalities are far too diverse, as are the events of each day. What can offer hope, however, is shifting from a focus of trying to say or do the "right" thing toward bringing our attention to the way we enter the moment; to "being with" the person who has dementia and focusing on a caring, compassionate connection wherever she is.

The essential first step remains the same. Take a slow, deep breath, and allow tensions, worries, or concerns to slip away with the exhale. By slowing ourselves down and focusing on being as relaxed and open as possible, we are more capable of creatively stretching beyond our traditional response to questions and more available to join the person who has dementia wherever she is in that moment. The goal is to listen to what the person with dementia is expressing, even behind the words.

In *Inside Alzheimer's* (2011), I write about a personal turning point when watching staff orient 98-year-old Maurice to the reality that the mother he was asking for died many years ago. Each time staff told Maurice our truth about his mother's death, the news was brand new from Maurice's perspective. Each time he grieved deeply and was inconsolable for the rest of the day, often not even remembering why he was so upset. After each time, he forgot the information and asked for his mother again. It seemed cruel to continually orient him to the reality of his mother's death when he was simply not able to retain the information or to process it over time. This situation required us to be flexible and creative in each interaction.

What we found to be effective was entering Maurice's world in the moment to get a sense of his emotion, and to try to discover what was behind his asking for his mother. When he was sad and missing his mother's company, we would ask questions that encouraged him to tell us about her and to relive some wonderful memories. Some days he was content with our simple companionship; other days he responded well when we shared how we missed being with our own mothers. When Maurice was worried or concerned for his mother's welfare, those of us who believed in life after death could confidently reassure him that his mother was very safe and doing well. When Maurice was upset because he needed his mother to do something for him, we let him know she could not be there at that time, but that we could certainly help him. Each occasion brought a new emotion, a new exploration, and a new connection with this tender, deeply feeling man. Maurice's questioning became less repetitive as we validated his emotions and provided comfort, familiarity, and safety.

We also began to notice a pattern; Maurice most consistently asked about his mother about one hour after lunch. We found that the upsetting search-and-questioning could be diverted on most days if we gave him some one-to-one time and included him in a therapeutic activity. For instance, listening to music from the Big Band era was particularly effective in connecting Maurice to positive memories.

The deceased may still be very much alive in the world of the person who has dementia, who may even report having seen and talked with the deceased recently. Challenging his reality is rarely productive. If these perceived interactions are highly upsetting to the person with dementia, he or she may be hallucinating and medications may be appropriate. I do encourage, however, entertaining the possibility that within these visions may be an opportunity to talk about the relationship with the deceased (to the degree possible) and to review life experiences and possible unresolved conflicts. The potential for reexamination and integration exists on some level when we reflect the core emotions and authentically identify with his or her experience. Our job is to be with the persons with dementia in whatever moment they are in and to let them know that they are not alone.

It is okay to talk about the deceased (perhaps even in the past tense) and to express some of your own emotions around the loss, as long as this is not upsetting to the person with dementia. Doing so has the potential to actively help the person with dementia through the grieving process. Bring pictures or play their favorite music to help reminisce about the person who has died. I have seen great healing and connections made with such sharing, with the person with dementia providing comfort with a gentle pat of the caregiver's hand or caress of the face. In those moments, each of you has some healing.

Only the person with dementia holds the key as to what is right in the moment. When we meet that person in his or her own reality, we become better able to encourage and respond to the emotional content behind the words or behaviors. When feelings are expressed and empathically reflected back to that person, he or she knows on some level he was heard and is not alone. It is the empathic and validating qualities of the relationship that offer the greatest potential for working through the challenging feelings behind the questioning.

What works in one moment may not work in the next. In trying to connect with a person who has dementia, we need to relax as much as possible and let go of our own frustrations, to be flexible with wherever the person takes us. This is not easy; it takes energy and clarity to remain creatively open. Particularly when the person with dementia is asking repetitive questions or has other challenging behaviors, it is important as professional caregivers to continually renew our own energy, maintain an awareness of the importance of taking care of ourselves, and allow in the support from others. Alzheimer's disease and related dementias present unique challenges; it is impossible for any one caregiver to do it all. Dementia care requires the participation of an entire community of people who are willing to become educated about the disease and take steps to explore the experiences of persons with dementia, even in grief. With each step taken, we open our hearts and show that there is hope that we can create a more compassionate, supportive network of care for everyone.

Nancy Pearce, MSW, LISW-CP, MS, is a licensed gerontological social worker with 30 years of experience working in long-term healthcare and hospice settings. She received an MS in Education from Syracuse University and a Master's in Social Work from the University of Connecticut. In her practice, she integrates her educational research foundations with understandings from both her work experience and studies in spiritual and religious wisdom traditions. Ms. Pearce specializes in working with persons who have dementia and teaches families, friends, and professionals, both nationally and internationally, how to communicate and connect effectively with persons with dementia, regardless of how advanced the dementia, and to co-create a more supportive community of care. She revised her top-selling book Inside Alzheimer's *(Forrason Press, 2011) and is a frequent contributor to* Social Work Today *and other publications.*

References

Childre, D., & Martin, H. (1999). *The HeartMath Solution.* San Francisco, CA: Harper Collins Publishers.

Childre, D., & Rozman, D. (2005). *Transforming Stress: The HeartMath Solution for Relieving Worry, Fatigue, and Tension.* Oakland, CA: New Harbinger Publications, Inc.

Miller, J. B., & Stiver, I. P. (1997). *The Healing Connections: How Women Form Relationships in Therapy and in Life.* Boston, MA: Beacon Press.

Pearce, N. (2011). *Inside Alzheimer's: How to Hear and Honor Connections with a Person who has Dementia.* Taylors, SC: Forrason Press.

CHAPTER 2

Voices
Still Here, Wherever Here Is

Elizabeth Uppman

It's best to keep the washcloth away from Grandma. If she gets hold of it, sitting on her bath chair, she'll dab the washcloth around her arms and legs and consider herself done. She is not done. I have to wash her armpits, hidden in folds of skin like layers of soft dough, her horny feet with their hard yellow toenails, and her bottom and crotch.

At first I expected her to be embarrassed that her granddaughter, whose diapers she once changed, is now washing her private parts. But she is unfazed, even cooperative. She has always been a genial person, acquiescent, happy to please. A photo from her honeymoon trip to Yellowstone shows an old-fashioned car with her on one side and a bear on the other, its nose through the window. My grandmother has a naughty, gleeful look on her face, but the bear just looks hungry. I imagine my grandfather holding the camera and pointing ("Go on up there, Mabel! He won't hurt you!"), and my grandmother, oblivious to the dismay this photo would cause her descendants some 60 years hence, mincing across the road to stand by the car, giggling. Like I said, she's acquiescent.

So besides maintaining control of the washcloth, the only other bathtime problem is the obvious one: friction, and its absence. I watch her lean and reach and try not to imagine what would happen to that mottled, tentative flesh if it hit porcelain suddenly, at high speed.

My grandmother is 98 years old. She doesn't use a wheelchair, walker, cane, or even orthopedic shoes. Her daily meds consist of a vitamin pill and an aspirin, to guard against stroke. She's healthy as a horse except for her mind. More than a decade now since her

Alzheimer's diagnosis, her memory, both short-term and long-term, is almost gone. I picture her memory as a slowly self-erasing blackboard containing names, images, references, and lots of shadowy words and phrases in a language that's increasingly foreign to her.

I bathe my grandmother and do other caregiving chores when my parents, with whom she lives, go out of town or out for an evening. This arrangement allows me to feel good that I'm helping out in the family without getting grossed-out or bogged down in the thanklessness of caregiving. I don't know if I'd be able to treat Grandma gently and with love if I had to be with her every hour of every day. Everyone tells my mom they don't know how she does it. I don't know, either.

I always think I will be serene and helpful when I stay with my grandmother, and I usually end up wanting to spank her. It's like Chinese water torture, the pointless questions and commentaries, the same ones over and over. It's like running a marathon on a quarter-mile track, round and round and nobody even wins.

Grandma often uncannily remembers the things you wish she'd forget. She cannot remember whose house this is, but she can remember that my mom, Marilyn, is supposed to return in two hours. These spots of clarity make for screamingly frustrating conversations. "Now, they're coming for me tonight?" she'll say.

"No, nobody's coming for you."

"But you brought me here, this afternoon."

"No, I didn't bring you, Grandma. You've been here the whole time." A pause, painful and confused. She tries again. "Who's coming?"

"Marilyn and Jerry are coming."

"And they'll come here?"

"Yes."

"You're sure?"

"Yes, I'm sure."

"Because maybe, do you think they might think we're at your house and go over there?"

"No, Grandma, they know we're here."

"Oh. You told them we're here?"

"No, Marilyn asked me to be here. She asked me to stay here with you, so I'm here."

"So Marilyn's coming?"

"Yes."

"And then she and I'll go home."

"No, Grandma, you'll stay here. This is your home."

"Oh, I don't know." A wry shake of her head. "We'll have to talk about that."

A longish pause. "So you're sure they're coming?"

"Yes, Grandma."

"Did they tell you they'd be coming here?"

"They live here. This is their house. They'll come back here."

"Oh. And then I'll go home with you."

"No, Grandma, you live here. This is your home."

A benevolent smile, to humor me. "Oh, no, that can't be right." Another pause. "When will they be here?"

"Soon." I try to smile at her.

"Now, you're sure they know we're here? Because maybe they'll think you and I are over at your house and then go over there."

"No, Grandma, I'm sure they'll come here."

"You're sure?"

This can go on for hours if I let it. The amazing part is, after rounds and rounds of questions and answers, after the fretting, the anxiety, the growing conviction that she's been improperly left here, wherever here is—after all this, you'd think the glorious arrival of my parents would be a cause for celebration and relief. But when they arrive, Grandma usually sits passively in her chair. She might not even smile.

It's situations like this that push caregiving beyond difficult to corrosive. The boring, repetitive, and often distasteful physical tasks (scrubbing dentures, wrestling with seat belts, wheedling her into clothes) are hard enough without the constant nagging questions. You try everything you can think of to reassure her and make her comfortable, but it's never enough.

I have a few coping strategies. I often pretend my conversations with Grandma are being broadcast live on NPR. I imagine Grandma's querulous, repetitive questions coming out of somebody's car stereo, and try to fashion the kind of replies that will impress listeners with my sublime patience and loving faithfulness.

When the NPR thing seems stupid, I think of the episode of "ER" where the earnest doctor dying of a brain tumor tells his teenaged daughter that the most important thing is generosity. Be generous with your time, your talent, yourself, he says, and I try to remember how little that generosity costs me, remembering that I'm big enough and calm enough to smile at Grandma instead of blowing her off or yelling at her. I try to remember that I have a choice.

When NPR and generosity both fail, I think about the yoga mantra that I sometimes apply, like a heating pad, when I'm feeling stressed: Be in the now moment. It's not about being able to do this for two weeks or two months or the rest of my life; it's about being able to do this right now, this moment.

And, since none of these strategies works 100 percent of the time, I buy myself a lot of chocolate.

On one long stay with Grandma, I moved my family into my parents' house, the house I grew up in, where Grandma now lives. I remember flying through one busy morning, trying to get the baby girl dressed on the bed in the guest room. She hid in the sheets, playing peek-a-boo. She looked up at me, crinkling her nose, and I suddenly saw that my hurry—my need to get all this stuff done and out of the way—was almost brutal, or at least unnecessary. So I stopped and blew a raspberry on her springy, taffy-colored tummy. She squealed with delight, and I remembered a moment years ago when Grandma and I stood in this same room. We were supposed to be polishing the furniture or putting things away, but I had found a book of song lyrics—show tunes and war songs, old songs from her times—which we leafed through, standing at the dresser in front of the big mirror. Grandma sang the ones she knew, her trombone-y old voice slooping up to the high notes and sliding down the low ones. She sang "Abba Dabba" and "Five Foot Two" and "Moon River." It made her laugh, and she turned the page to find the next one, playing hooky from the day, with me her accomplice, her partner in mischief.

I felt that same joy with the baby on the bed that morning—a stolen piece of fun plucked from the grinding gears of the morning's relentless time clock. And I realized something: Grandma would have liked to play with this baby. Grandma should be here.

But she isn't here, in any but the most superficial sense. She is lost.

My grandmother usually seems little and fragile, her steps like a bird's, her movements tentative and deflective. But sometimes, like when I give her a bath or when I wake her up, she seems huge: flesh hanging off arms and collarbones, unending folds of belly and thigh.

Caring for an Alzheimer's patient is a lot like caring for a baby: you monitor her meals, you tie her shoelaces. But the soul of the task is different. While my baby girl always knows who's in charge—me—my grandmother has her doubts. To her I am still a whippersnapper. She can never quite believe I'm old enough or smart enough to get us all through the day. Her lingering belief in herself as the competent one compels me to keep up the slight fiction that I'm helping her, not controlling her. Besides, when I pretend I'm only giving her advice and guidance, then I can believe she's still fundamentally okay. I don't want her to be helpless, I want her to be help-able.

Caring for Grandma always makes me think about her death. When I stay overnight with her, I mount the stairs in the morning to wake her up, imagining I might find a dead body instead of a grandmother in the bed. It would be terrible and it would be a terrible relief. I must correct myself: It will be terrible when it happens in the coming months or years. And it will be a terrible relief.

Of course, she might not go easy, in her sleep. She might put up a fight. People can lose almost everything and still continue to live, bedridden, incontinent, incapable of speech. My grandmother might end up like that. The fact that there's nothing wrong with her 98-year-old body seems like a miracle except when it seems like a curse.

I often wonder how aware Grandma is of her mind's creeping deterioration. If at some point you began to perceive that the you-ness of you were disappearing, wouldn't you panic? I don't see panic in Grandma—not anymore. Once, several years ago, when she was supposed to be asleep, I overheard her reciting, in the darkness of the bedroom, a litany of self-identity: "My husband is Archie. My children are Bob, Marilyn, and Jim. We live in New Salem." She may have been battling back the fear of losing those names and places, or she may have just been putting herself to sleep. I don't know.

For awhile at the beginning of her dementia it was obvious when she knew or suspected something wasn't right, like when nobody would allow her to help with the dinner dishes or hold the baby. Those limits frustrated her, but she was too polite to complain. Nowadays she seems more and more oblivious, and for that I'm frankly grateful. If she is going to cling to her life this tenaciously, I would like for her to find a way to absent herself from its indignities and pain. I hope the spark of selfness that makes Grandma Grandma burns out before her body does, so that the final days and hours of suffering are just a biological end-game, just a brute process that works itself out the way it needs to. I hope she doesn't have to stick around for all that.

One morning Grandma was particularly agitated as I drove her to the Club, the adult day-care facility she attends three days a week. She wouldn't have been so upset if she hadn't been amazingly in command of a few important facts: I was taking her there—to this slightly familiar place—but I wasn't staying, and after a certain amount of time I would come pick her up. All of this could only mean it was some kind of holding-pen or way-station or, worse, school. (Grandma started school not knowing a word of English with a teacher who, according to the family stories, was just plain mean.)

"Well, am I supposed to—" She made a vague gesture, "...supposed to *learn* something there?"

"Well, you'll play bingo and have a nice lunch—"

"What?"

"Bingo," I said loudly. "And a nice lunch."

This only confirmed her fears. She shook her head. "Well, I'm sorry to put you through this. I'm sorry you have to do all this."

And there it was, the glimpse, ever so small, of my old Grandma, the one who paid her own way, who made herself small, who wouldn't trouble anyone to open a tight jar or give her a ride to the store in the snow. My old Grandma, the one I knew, would apologize that I had to wash her and dress her and take her to day care. She would feel bad that she was such an inconvenience to me.

I found nothing to say in reply, none of the jolly stock phrases or mollifying comments or veiled cajolings that make up most of our conversation nowadays. We drove in silence over a bridge, past a hedge. It wasn't until days later that I thought of an appropriate reply, and then, of course, it was too late to say it. But what I would have liked to say to her is, "I'm sorry too, Grandma."

Elizabeth Uppman is a writer living in Overland Park, Kansas. Her essays and poems have appeared in Good Housekeeping; salon.com; Brain, Child; Tango; The Kansas City Star; *and in various Hospice Foundation of America publications. She has a BA in English from Carleton College. She is currently working on a memoir.*

Editor's Note: This essay was originally published in K. J. Doka (Ed.), Living with grief: Alzheimer's disease *(pp. 127–133). Washington, DC: Hospice Foundation of America.*

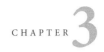

And I have lost him twice: Grief in Dementia Caregivers

Katherine P. Supiano

> *"I never loved but one man in my life*
> *and I have lost him twice."*

In this quote from Edmond Rostand's *Cyrano de Bergerac*, the heroine Roxanne voices her realization that she loves the homely musketeer Cyrano, not the dashing Christian. Her awareness comes as Cyrano is dying and his words reveal his love for her, words he had composed on Christian's behalf and allowed him to speak to Roxanne. A retired English professor, in a caregiver support group I facilitated, shared these words as he described his wife's cognitive deterioration and his love for her despite dramatic changes in her personality. The quote captured the essence of both his present and eventual bereavement as a dementia caregiver.

In the 30-plus years since this gentleman was in my caregiver support group, much has changed in our awareness of Alzheimer's disease and other dementias. Amazing advances have taken place in early diagnosis, psychobehavioral interventions, and development of vital support services, but the caregiving experience remains much the same. It is a caregiving journey marked by progressive loss and multiple griefs.

THE CAREGIVING JOURNEY TO GRIEF

Family caregiving in all its forms is challenging and often described as *burden*. The term "burden" reflects the reality and magnitude of the tasks and their associated responsibilities and, in and of itself, is neither bad nor good; it is a usual component of human relationships and the giving and receiving of care. In the context of dementia caregiving, the unique features of the disease add a considerable layer of difficulty. Many persons with memory loss experience delays in getting the correct diagnosis, resulting in frustration, fear, and diminished trust within families and with healthcare providers. Memory loss is frequently mistaken for normal aging, minimized or hidden by those affected, or ascribed to stress or other life circumstances. Early symptoms of memory loss or behavior change are often misattributed to personality characteristics: "He never pays attention," "He doesn't care," "She has always been this way." Even with diagnostic clarity, it is difficult for caregivers not to take behavioral symptoms personally, especially symptoms like paranoia and combativeness. As is the case with thought disorders and mood disorders, caregivers of those with cognitive disorders have a hard time separating the person from the disease. Unlike caregiving in other disease processes such as cancer or heart disease, the care transaction may be interpreted as being underappreciated by the care recipient.

The trajectory of Alzheimer's disease and most dementias is measured in decades. Over the length of the Alzheimer's disease process, a care recipient may require round-the-clock care for 4 to 7 years. Thirty-one percent of active dementia caregivers in the United States have been caregiving for over 5 years; 15% have been caregiving for over 10 years (National Alliance for Caregiving (NAC), 2009, p. 20).

Dementia caregiving is physically demanding. On average, caregivers spend over 20 hours per week providing assistance with activities of daily living, including dressing, bathing, and mobility (NAC, 2009, p. 21). Caregivers who live with the care recipient frequently experience sleep disturbances that can persist long after caregiving transitions, such as care facility placement or death of the care recipient.

Dementia caregiving is also emotionally demanding, with 31% of caregivers reporting high levels of stress (NAC, 2009, p. 50). Over time, caregivers may become less engaged in their own self-care and increasingly vulnerable to illness, fatigue, and psychological depletion. Following a similar pattern, caregivers report less social engagement, with 53% reporting that caregiving reduces available time with friends and other family members (NAC, 2009, p. 51). Caregivers, particularly female caregivers, often reduce their employment or withdraw from the workforce, placing their financial security and employment advancement at risk (Alzheimer's Association, 2014). Community services may be unavailable or expensive, and obtaining and maintaining support services can be frustrating and time-consuming.

Among these many challenges, changes in the memory and personality of the care recipient loom largest. Most caregivers work diligently to "find the person within the disease," respecting past preferences while creatively responding to emerging symptoms with patience and forbearance. Much of our personality and our ability to recognize and interact with those we love are located within memory. Memory decline robs the person of the self and diminishes the capacity for relational engagement. This is the essence of losing the beloved twice: once when the loved one is unable to engage and again when the person physically dies.

HELPING DEMENTIA CAREGIVERS PRIOR TO THE DEATH OF A LOVED ONE

As with all chronic, progressive diseases, early diagnosis adds immeasurably to the exploration of care options and the development of a flexible care plan. Early diagnosis optimizes education of the patient and family, allowing them to develop a professional support team that, ideally, includes the neurologist, primary care provider, social worker, and health educator, paving the way for introduction of community supports. Patient and family education, such as that available from the Alzheimer's Association, provides essential information about the disease trajectory and symptoms that can help patients and families understand the process and prepare for typical transitions of care. Early education is critical in those dementias that have very difficult symptoms and behaviors such as Lewy body dementia (LBD) and frontotemporal dementia (FTD).

Advance care planning is vital in the care of those with cognitive impairment, as diminished capacity is a certain eventuality. Advance care planning includes both discussions with medical providers for health-specific information and with family members about patient preferences and goals of care. Most states have advance care plan documents including healthcare proxy/medical decision-maker forms, advance directives (sometimes called "living wills"), and Physician Orders for Life-Sustaining Treatment (POLST) forms or Medical Orders for Life-Sustaining Treatment (MOLST) forms. The forms and documentation are important, but it is the conversations that allow the person with early-stage dementia to express goals, preferences, and wishes that contribute most to a clear understanding of the care setting and treatment interventions that are preferred. In addition, these conversations begin a process where the patient and family speak openly about the situation, and family members have the opportunity to express support in honoring and understanding the patient's wishes. Plans about who will participate in the care can also be discussed; shared family caregiving mitigates the isolation that can become a debilitating component of dementia caregiving. Timely family communication that is open and honest fosters the continuation of social relationships outside the family, particularly with friends, who may be aware that "something" is going on, but may be hesitant to express concerns and offer support.

In addition to these informal supports, open communication paves the way for appropriate acquisition of formal supports. Involvement in dementia caregiver support groups and support groups for early-stage care recipients is beneficial for social engagement and information sharing. Community services such as supported transportation, cognitive stimulation programs in senior centers, exercise programs, respite care, and adult day care are relatively low-cost and delay institutional placement. Early introduction of services reduces the risk that caregivers will become "lone rangers" who are reluctant to utilize services, apprehensive that no one can help the care recipient as well as they do.

Several novel interventions have been developed to equip caregivers to understand and effectively respond to difficult symptoms and behaviors in care recipients. Among the interventions that have been tested in multi-site national trials are Resources for Enhancing Alzheimer's Caregiver Health (REACH-II) (Gitlin, Winter, Dennis, Hodgson, & Hauck, 2010) and the New York University Caregiver Intervention (Mittelman, Epstein, & Pierzchala, 2003; Gaugler, Roth, Haley, & Mittelman, 2008). These interventions use multiple structured approaches including individual caregiver consultation, family strategy sessions, and ongoing guidance and support. Several of these interventions have demonstrated improved caregiver health and lower levels of caregiver depression and stress, and delayed nursing home placement of the care recipient.

Professional care providers have much to offer caregivers in the early and middle stages of dementia. They can support the caregiver-care recipient relationship at all levels: the past, through reminiscence, addressing old hurts and facilitating forgiveness; the present, with managing day-to-day challenges; and the future, by encouraging important conversations and preparing for the death of the care recipient. Professional care providers must accurately assess the coping skills of caregivers and encourage self-care. It is essential that professional care providers take a detailed loss inventory. Asking questions such as, "Up until the time of the death, what was the most challenging loss you faced?" or, "How did you cope with past losses?" can yield essential information on coping style and ability. Providers must also carefully monitor caregivers for depression, anxiety, and sleep disturbances.

The demands of dementia caregiving contribute to the eventual bereavement experience, but situational factors can also impact grief. Caregivers with multiple caregiving responsibilities (parents, in-laws, children with special needs) are burdened with competing demands. At the time of the care recipient's death, the caregiver may not be able to grieve fully, but must immediately attend to other family members in need, often being placed in the role of "the strong one." The circumstances of the death may predispose caregivers to poor bereavement outcomes: being absent at the time of death; being present at the time of death but perceiving the experience as a "bad" death; or being present for the death but without other people there for support. An underrecognized phenomenon is "acute-on-chronic death." In this situation, the caregiver is prepared for a gradual dying process from dementia, but the care recipient dies a sudden death, such as from a fall or aspiration event. The caregiver then grieves the decline associated with progressive dementia, but must also reconcile to an unforeseen trauma.

A final variable is the availability of both formal and informal supports for dementia caregiving. Social supports may be available, but of poor quality. High quality supports, when available, may not be utilized by caregivers for a variety of reasons including pride, denial of need, independence, or embarrassment about or on behalf of the care recipient. Similarly, community resources may not be available, of poor quality, or too expensive; high quality, suitably-priced resources may not be utilized by some caregivers just as social supports are underutilized. Lack of supports for any of these reasons may undermine the caregiver and impact bereavement outcome.

WHEN DEATH COMES

According to Boerner and Schulz (2009), there are three perspectives on dementia caregiver grief. The first originates from a cumulative stress perspective; the burden of caregiving followed by the death depletes the caregiver's available resources to address grief, leading to difficult adjustment. In contrast, the second perspective argues that stress is reduced when the care recipient dies, bringing relief and an easier grief process. The third perspective contends that because caregivers can anticipate the dementia death, they can prepare for it (by planning ahead, saying goodbye, getting affairs in order) and ease into a grief transition. One can easily imagine a single caregiver's grief falling largely into one of these three categories, depending on circumstances. A combination of these perspectives being voiced by a single caregiver would not be inconceivable. Each perspective makes sense in some situations; what might account for these differing experiences?

Although painful, grief is among the most natural of human conditions and most people grieve well with coping skills, social support, and time. In fact, the majority of bereaved dementia caregivers do realize a positive and adaptive grief process, and return to pre-caregiving levels of function and socialization (Boerner & Schulz, 2009; Givens, Prigerson, Kiely, Shaffer, & Mitchell, 2011; Shear, 2012). There are some distinctive features about losing someone to dementia that are frequently expressed by bereaved caregivers.

Caregivers have not only lost the object of their care, they have lost a role and a purpose for living. This reality can result in an unsettled state when figuring out how to use personal time to reestablish social connections, and finding a new purpose in life after years of caregiving.

It is very common in the initial days and weeks of acute grief for grievers in all death circumstances to feel doubt and even guilt about the dying process and the death. For bereaved dementia caregivers at this time in grief, well-intended accolades of devoted caregiving may ring hollow.

Those grieving the death of a person with dementia often experience *disenfranchised grief* (Doka, 2008), grief that is not socially endorsed. Bereaved dementia caregivers are often told, by well-meaning people, to be happy that their family member's suffering is over and that they are now free to enjoy themselves again. These statements can be dismissive of the real feelings of missing the person, either near the end of life or in earlier years.

WHEN GRIEF BECOMES COMPLICATED

While rewarding for many, caring for a person with Alzheimer's disease is challenging and can have deleterious health and mental health effects. For 10-20% of caregivers (Kersting, Brahler, Glaesmer, & Wagner, 2001; Middleton, Burnett, Raphael, & Martinek, 1996), these effects persist into bereavement in the form of complicated grief, termed "Persistent Complex Bereavement Disorder" in *The Diagnostic and Statistical Manual of Mental Disorders* (5th ed.; *DSM-5;* American Psychiatric Association, 2013). Unlike grief that progresses toward a resolved, integrated status, complicated grief is characterized by unabated maladaptive thoughts, feelings, and behaviors that obstruct adjustment. Complicated grief is a state of chronic mourning that includes persistent yearning, recurrent intrusive thoughts of the person who died, preoccupation with sorrow including ruminative thoughts, excessive bitterness, alienation from previous social relationships, difficulty accepting the death, and perceived purposelessness of life. These symptoms contribute to profound social, occupational, and functional disturbance (Boelen & Prigerson, 2012).

Bereaved dementia caregivers have unique risk factors that may contribute to complicated grief. Dementia caregiving requires ongoing adjustment within the caregiver-care recipient dyad, particularly as the caregiver prepares for the loss of this significant relationship (Noyes et al., 2010; Lewis, Hepburn, Narayan, & Kirk, 2005). An inability to accommodate relationship change and the eventual death of the care recipient may predict ineffective post-death integration of grief (Piiparinen & Whitlatch, 2011; Sanders & Corley, 2003; Holland, Futtermans, Thompson, Moran, & Gallagher-Thompson, 2013). Caregivers with insecure attachment patterns are at risk for complicated grief upon the death of the care recipient (Mikulincer & Shaver, 2008), as attachment patterns are moderated over time by the quality of the relationship between the griever and the deceased (Mancini, Robinaugh, Shear, & Bonanno, 2009).

Other reported complicated grief risk factors in dementia caregivers include: positive view of the caregiving role, perceived gratifying communication with the care recipient, high expressed affection by the caregiver, and high perceived caregiving burden (Schulz, Boerner, Shear, Zhang, & Gitlin, 2006). In an interesting finding from the national REACH study of Alzheimer's disease caregivers, 23% of caregivers indicated they were "not prepared" for the death (Hebert,

Dang, & Schulz, 2006), and this was highly associated with complicated grief. Dementia caregiving is also associated with depression and anxiety, known risk factors for complicated grief (Barry, Kasl, & Prigerson, 2002; Keyes et al., 2014).

Bereaved caregivers with complicated grief feel stuck; they feel that life is moving on and they are not. They may have strong feelings of longing for the deceased care recipient, self-doubt at decisions made on behalf of the care recipient, guilt for words spoken or for nursing home placement, anger at the disease or family members, or regret. Sometimes they feel that others have "pulled away" from them, or were absent at critical times. They may feel removed from others they once enjoyed and unable to resume those relationships. While many bereaved caregivers may experience some of these thoughts and feelings, they typically dissipate with time and support. Pervasive and unrelenting yearning and feelings of guilt, failure, and shame, and deteriorating social relationships suggest a complicated grief process that merits special care.

Several national multi-site dementia caregiver studies have reported complicated grief in bereaved caregivers and called for treatment and prevention strategies to mitigate poor bereavement outcomes and enhance healthy grief in caregivers following the death of a care recipient (Schulz, Boerner, Shear, Zhang, & Gitlin, 2006).

For the minority of persons unable to effectively grieve, specialized treatment for complicated grief and comorbid conditions can restore a healthy grief process (Shear, 2012). Prior research has supported the need for targeted interventions to address complicated grief (Shear et al., 2011). One demonstrated treatment for complicated grief, developed by Katherine Shear and colleagues (2005, 2014) is Complicated Grief Therapy (CGT), a manualized treatment protocol applied in individual psychotherapy, involving phases of psychoeducation, application of dual-process (loss and restoration) approaches, focused attention on trauma-like symptoms, revisiting of the relationship with the deceased, and planning for the future. CGT has been adapted as a group psychotherapy intervention (Supiano & Luptak, 2014) and has been found to be effective in older adults with complicated grief. Complicated grief group therapy is presently being evaluated in bereaved dementia caregivers who meet criteria for complicated grief (Supiano, study ongoing).

Rather than regarding complicated grief through the earlier lens of "pathological grief, " the aim of these therapeutic approaches is to restore a healthy grief process that leads to "integrated grief" (Shear, 2012), allowing the griever to move into a new life with satisfying relationships and purpose, informed by a realistic remembrance of the one who died.

CONCLUSION

Caring for a person with dementia is both demanding and potentially rewarding; for many caregivers, it represents the fulfillment of promised affection and commitment. There are presently 15 million dementia caregivers in the United States (Alzheimer's Association, 2014, p. 30), each facing multiple losses, challenges, and daily small, but inevitable, griefs. The devotion of these caregivers merits interpersonal support and societal regard. Compassionately guiding persons with dementia and their caregivers on this journey requires acknowledgment of the eventual death of the care recipient. Prompt and accurate diagnosis, advance care planning, education, support, and resources may not alter the disease course, but can smooth transitions of care, foster dignity, respect the voice of the care recipient, and enhance the grief and mourning of the family and friends.

Recognizing that persons with dementia are indeed twice lost, we can offer recognition of the person within the dementia at all stages of the disease. Just as the professor in my caregiver support group realized, the beloved is always with us. Modeling this awareness in our service to caregivers may enable them to navigate the personality changes and trials of caregiving in a way that honors the care recipient and, when the time of death comes, facilitates healthy grief in caregivers.

Katherine P. Supiano, PhD, LCSW, FT, F-GSA, is an associate professor in the College of Nursing, and the director of the Caring Connections: A Hope and Comfort in Grief *program, at the University of Utah. Dr. Supiano's research is in clinical interventions in complicated grief, suicide survivorship, and prison hospice. She has been a practicing clinical social worker and psychotherapist for over 30 years. Her clinical practice has included care of older adults with depression and multiple chronic health concerns, family therapy, end-of-life care, and bereavement care. Dr. Supiano is a Fellow in the Gerontological Society of America, a Fellow of Thanatology, and a founding member of the Social Work Hospice and*

Palliative Care Network. She received her PhD in Social Work at the University of Utah as a John A. Hartford Foundation Doctoral Fellow.

REFERENCES

Alzheimer's Association. (2014). Alzheimer's disease facts and figures. *Alzheimer's & Dementia, 10*(2), 1-80.

American Psychiatric Association. (2013). *Diagnostic and statistical manual of mental disorders (5th edition).* Arlington, VA: American Psychiatric Publishing.

Barry, L. C., Kasl, S. V., & Prigerson, H. G. (2002). Psychiatric disorders among bereaved persons: The role of perceived circumstances of death and preparedness for death. *American Journal of Geriatric Psychiatry, 10*(4), 447-457.

Boelen, P. A., & Prigerson, H. G. (2012). Commentary on the inclusion of persistent complex bereavement-related disorder in DSM-5. *Death Studies, 36*(9), 771-794.

Boerner, K., & Schulz, R. (2009). Caregiving, bereavement and complicated grief. *Bereavement Care: For All Those Who Help the Bereaved, 28*(3), 10-13. doi: 10.1080/02682620903355382

Chiu, Y. C., Lee, Y. N., Wang, P. C., Chang, T. H., Li, C. L., Hsu, W. C., & Lee, S. H. (2014). Family caregivers' sleep disturbance and its associations with multilevel stressors when caring for patients with dementia. *Aging & Mental Health, 18*(1), 92-101. doi: 10.1080/13607863.2013.837141

Doka, K. J. (2008). Disenfranchised grief in historical and cultural perspective. In M. S. Stroebe, R. O. Hansson, W. Stroebe, & H. Schut (Eds.), *Handbook of bereavement research and practice: Advances in theory and intervention* (pp. 223-240). Washington, DC: American Psychological Association.

Gaugler, J. E., Roth, D. L., Haley, W. E., Mittelman, M. S. (2008). Can counseling and support reduce burden and depressive symptoms in caregivers of people with Alzheimer's disease during the transition to institutionalization? Results from the New York University Caregiver Intervention Study. *Journal of the American Geriatrics Society,* 56:421–8.

Givens, J. L., Prigerson, H. G., Kiely, D. K., Shaffer, M. L., & Mitchell, S. L. (2011). Grief among family members of nursing home residents with advanced dementia. *The American Journal of Geriatric Psychiatry, 19*(6), 543-550. doi: 10.1097/JGP.0b013e31820dcbe0

Gitlin, L. N., Winter, L., Dennis, M. P., Hodgson, N., & Hauck, W. W. (2010). Targeting and managing behavioral symptoms in individuals with dementia: A randomized trial of a nonpharmacological intervention. *Journal of the American Geriatrics Society*, 58:1465–74.

Hebert, R. S., Dang, Q., & Schulz, R. (2006). Preparedness for the death of a loved one and mental health in bereaved caregivers of patients with dementia: Findings from the REACH study. *Journal of Palliative Medicine, 9*(3), 683-693. doi: 10.1089/jpm.2006.9.683

Holland, J. M., Futtermans, A., Thompson, L. W., Moran, C., & Gallagher-Thompson, D. (2013). Difficulties accepting the loss of a spouse: A precursor for intensified grieving among widowed older adults. *Death Studies, 37*, 126-144.

Kersting, A., Brahler, E., Glaesmer, H., & Wagner, B. (2011). Prevalences of complicated grief in a representative population-based sample. *Journal of Affective Disorders, 131*, 339-343.

Keyes, K. M., Pratt, C., Galea, S., McLaughlin, K. A., Koenen, K. C., & Shear, M. K. (2014). The burden of loss: Unexpected death of a loved one and psychiatric disorders across the life course in a national study. *The American Journal of Psychiatry, 171*(8), 864-871. doi: 10.1176/appi.ajp.2014.13081132

Lewis, M. L., Hepburn, K., Narayan, S., & Kirk, L. N. (2005). Relationship matters in dementia caregiving. *American Journal of Alzheimer's Disease and Other Dementias, 20*(6), 341-347.

Mancini, A. D., Robinaugh, A. D., Shear, K., & Bonanno, G. A. (2009). Does attachment avoidance help people cope with loss? The moderating effects of relationship quality. *Journal of Clinical Psychology, 65*, 1127–1136. doi:10.1002/jclp.20601

Middleton, W., Burnett, P., Raphael, B., & Martinek, N. (1996). The bereavement response: A cluster analysis. *British Journal of Psychiatry, 169*(2), 167-171.

Mikulincer, M., & Shaver, P. R. (2008). An attachment perspective on bereavement. In M. S. Stroebe, R. O. Hansson, H. Schut, & W. Stroebe (Eds.), *Handbook of bereavement research and practice: Advances in theory and intervention* (pp. 87–112). Washington, DC: American Psychological Association.

Mittelman, M. S., Epstein, C., & Pierzchala, A. (2003). *Counseling the Alzheimer's caregiver: A resource for health care professionals.* Chicago, IL: AMA Press.

National Alliance for Caregiving (2009). Caregiving in the US. Retrieved from http://www.caregiving.org/data/Caregiving_in_the_US_2009_full_report.pdf

Noyes, B. B., Hill, R. D., Hicken, B. L., Luptak, M., Rupper, R., Dailey, N. K., & Bair, B. D. (2010). Review: The role of grief in dementia caregiving. *American Journal of Alzheimer's Disease and Other Dementias, 25*(9), 9-17.

Piiparinen, R., & Whitlatch, C. J. (2011). Existential loss as a determinant to well-being in the dementia caregiving dyad: A conceptual model. *Dementia, 10*(2), 185-201.

Rostand, E. (1897/trans.1966). *Cyrano de Bergerac.* Translated by Brian Hocker. New York, NY: Bantam Books.

Sanders, S., & Corley, C. S. (2003). Are they grieving? A qualitative analysis examining grief in caregivers of individuals with Alzheimer's Disease. *Social Work in Health Care, 37*(3), 35-53.

Schulz, R., Boerner, K., Shear, K., Zhang, S., & Gitlin, L. N. (2006). Predictors of complicated grief among dementia caregivers: A prospective study of bereavement. *The American Journal of Geriatric Psychiatry, 14*, 650-658. doi:10.1097/01.JGP.0000203178.44894.db

Shear, K., Frank, E., Houck, P. R., & Reynolds, C. F. (2005). Treatment of complicated grief: A randomized controlled trial. *JAMA, 293*(21), 2601-2608. doi: 293/21/2601 10.1001/jama.293.21.2601

Shear, M. K., Simon, N., Wall, M., Zisook, S., Neimeyer, R., Duan, N., Reynolds, C., Lebowitz, B., Sung, N., Ghesquiere, A., Gorscak, B., Clayton, P., Ito, M., Nakajima, S., Konishi, T., Melhem, N., Meert, K., Schiff, M., O'Connor, M., Sareen, J., Bolton, J., Skritskaya, N., Mancini, A.D., & Keshaviah, A. (2011). Complicated grief and related bereavement issues for DSM-5. *Depression & Anxiety, 28*(2), 103-117.

Shear, M. K. (2012). Getting straight about grief. *Depression & Anxiety, 29*, 461-464. doi: 10.1002/da.211963

Shear, M., Wang, Y., Skritskaya, N., Duan, N., Mauro, C., Ghesquiere, A. (2014). Treatment of complicated grief in elderly persons: A randomized clinical trial. *JAMA Psychiatry*. Published online September 24, 2014. doi:10.1001/jamapsychiatry.2014.1242

Supiano, K. P., & Luptak, M. (2014). Complicated grief in older adults: A randomized controlled trial of complicated grief group therapy. *The Gerontologist, 54*(5), 840-856. doi: 10.1093/geront/gnt076

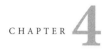

Voices
One Family's Encounters
with Dementia

Donna M. Corr and Charles A. Corr

A t the outset, Donna was not altogether comfortable with our plan to write this chapter. She says she is confident that what we have written would upset her mother. If so, Donna is concerned that Sadie may visit us one day from the "great beyond" to chastise us for sharing such private family matters in this way. In the end, however, we both have decided to write about encounters with dementia in our family in the hope that what we have written may offer some helpful lessons for others. Our temporary reluctance to write about these encounters perhaps reflects an underlying sense of embarrassment or shame, even though we know and urge others to realize that dementias of all types are biologically based and should not be matters of dishonor or humiliation; after all, no one voluntarily chooses to have cognitive impairment.

Encounters with dementia in our family span three generations: the first involving Donna's grandmother, Marie; the second involving Donna's mother and stepfather, Sadie and Jim; and the third involving Donna herself, and me. In these descriptions, we draw on factual information, memories from family members, and our own recollections.

As Donna and I have done so often over the years, this chapter is a product of our collaboration. For simplicity, we have chosen to identify Chuck in the first person singular ("I") and the two of us together in the first person plural ("we"). However, there should be no misunderstanding: This is *our* story.

Marie

In the early years of the 20th century, Marie and her husband Frank left Europe, "…to avoid Frank's having to serve in Kaiser Franz Josef's Bohemian ceremonial guard in the Austro-Hungarian Empire." They immigrated to the United States, settling on a humble farm in Hinckley, Ohio, south of Cleveland, where their four children were born. The family managed to get by, but it was a hard life on the farm. When they grew older, Marie and Frank sold the farm and moved to a small house in Cleveland.

Around the time of Frank's death, Marie began to display early symptoms of dementia. She had suffered from arthritis for many years, leaving Donna with vivid memories of the odor of the liniment Marie used while trying to moderate the pain in her joints. Marie's developing dementia compounded her health challenges. For example, Marie began to complain that a neighbor was crawling through a window and stealing the butterscotch candies she kept in a jar to snack on during the day. Her adult children, all of whom lived nearby, tried their best to care for Marie, but eventually she had to be settled in a long-term care facility. In time, she no longer recognized her children or grandchildren. One of our daughters has a clear memory of earlier conversations with her great-grandmother in English, but by the time Marie was relocated to long-term care, she spoke to our daughter only in Czech, a language our daughter did not speak. In fact, Marie seemed to think of herself as a young girl, back in what the family had always called Czechoslovakia.

While still mobile, Marie was confined in a locked ward for "wanderers," yet one day she did get out in a snow storm dressed only in her nightgown and slippers. Eventually, Marie was found a few blocks away sitting in a snow bank. While she did not do any harm to herself during this adventure, the episode shows how she remained strong physically, even as her mental faculties became increasingly compromised. Marie eventually was bedbound and unable to engage in typical interactions with others. She died peacefully at the age of 94.

Marie's dementia followed a familiar course: from early symptoms of confusion and loss of short-term memory, to inability to care for herself and reversion to a child-like status, to becoming unable to recognize family members, to being confined to her bed, and eventually to death. Marie's dementia demonstrated how this disease can take over an individual's personality resulting in increasingly odd behaviors, how ordinary interactions may become difficult or impossible, and how decisions may need to be made to relocate the person to a long-term care facility when family caregiving is no longer adequate to meet the immediate needs.

Sadie and Jim

Marie and Frank's oldest child, Sadie, met her future husband, Tony, when he and some friends came out to the farm on weekends to enjoy the chicken dinners the family prepared as a means of supplementing their income. Sadie and Tony married in 1932 and their only child, Donna, my future wife, was born a few years later. Tony worked in a factory all his life until he developed heart problems. He was treated at the Cleveland Clinic using the then-newly-developed technique of open heart surgery. Unfortunately, the results described a well-known path: successful surgery, development of an infection, and the patient's early death.

Sadie's widowhood at the age of 48 was not at all part of the life plan she had envisioned for herself. Sadie had always been a deeply religious person, heavily involved in numerous church activities. In her view, she had lived a good life, one in which she had more than met her familial and religious obligations. She felt cheated that such a life should have led to the untimely death of her husband, the first major loss she had experienced.

After Tony's death, Sadie endured a difficult bereavement. She had graduated from high school but like many women of her time, she had primarily been a homemaker and had no vocational training to start a career. She was fortunate that a friend helped her get a job.

When Sadie's only child, Donna, and I married in 1962, we moved to St. Louis where I was a graduate student in philosophy ("How could this guy ever expect to support you properly?" Tony often asked). With Donna gone, Sadie became more isolated in Cleveland.

Sadie and Donna (and I) exchanged visits between Cleveland and St. Louis as often as we could, and Sadie took delight in the births of our three children. But in many ways, Sadie was on her own in Cleveland. Her brother and two sisters had all married, but even a close relationship with one sister did not bring the companionship and support she had experienced in her own marriage.

Several years after Tony's death, almost in desperation, Sadie shared her difficulties with her family physician. He urged her to get out more, suggesting that she join a church group. Quite unexpectedly on the first night she attended the group, a man crossed the room to introduce himself. Like Sadie, Jim was widowed with grown children. He was a Navy veteran, handy with tools and practical matters, and a genial conversationalist. He had a good job and owned two houses.

Sadie and Jim married in January 1971. They enjoyed many happy years together and Sadie's second husband soon became a beloved "Uncle Jim" to our family.

But a dark cloud emerged when Jim's younger sister developed signs of early onset dementia in her mid-fifties and died not long afterwards. Unfortunately, the genetic implications of that diagnosis were borne out when Jim developed similar symptoms in the late 1980s.

As his still-undiagnosed disease progressed, Jim was admitted to a hospital in Cleveland; a month later, his diagnosis of Alzheimer's disease was confirmed. Subsequently, he was transferred to a long-term care facility near their home.

Throughout the lengthy course of Jim's illness, Sadie found it very difficult to accept what was happening to him (and to her) after experiencing her mother's dementia and Tony's death. In both the hospital and the long-term care facility, she visited Jim daily, bringing his favorite foods and applying lotion to his skin to try to keep him from developing bed sores. Sadie sought heroically to stave off the progression of Jim's disease and greatly dreaded the prospect of enduring Jim's death and having to cope once again with mourning a spouse. She could hardly bear to consider what she viewed as the grim possibilities she faced in the future, even though those prospects were always on her mind.

Donna and I visited Sadie and Jim whenever we could, but such visits were limited by our professional responsibilities (Donna as a nurse and I as a faculty member at Southern Illinois University Edwardsville), and the needs of our three growing children. On several occasions, Sadie and Jim came to St. Louis. Unfortunately, one time Jim's car ran off the road in eastern Illinois on their way to visit us. After that experience, they made the trip by air, but on another occasion, Jim wandered off while Sadie used the airport restroom. Happily, neither Jim nor Sadie suffered serious injury in the automobile accident (although their car was a total wreck), and Jim was soon found in the airport. But these two events were clear cautionary signs. They also reflected Sadie's tendency to challenge Jim to do things that were, by then, really beyond his capacities. This way of coping for Sadie resulted in part from her underlying anxieties, her strong personality, and her reluctance to accept how much things had changed for Jim.

It was difficult for all of us to witness the changes in Jim. For a man who always kept his tools and household implements in immaculate condition, it was disconcerting to realize one day that he did not recognize a simple screwdriver. On another day, it was hard to watch him holding a key, unable to determine how it was to be used to unlock a door in order to follow his habitual pattern of smoking his cigarettes outside the house. In the early years of his disease, Jim could recall many events from the distant past and carry on conversations with anyone he encountered in ways that concealed his increasing memory and intellectual deficits. Still, once while we were driving around the city, he asked, "What is that golden thing hanging in the sky this evening?" Having to identify the moon for him threw light on his emerging dementia, even if we still didn't know much about how to address this problem.

Perhaps my most vivid memory is of a night when Sadie and Jim were visiting our home in St. Louis. Jim became quite upset and angry at Sadie and Donna. We were puzzled over this unusual aggressive behavior in a person previously known only for his gentle demeanor. Jim knew something was wrong, but could only try to convey his distress to another male without making clear the assistance he required. It was only when he lost control of his bladder as we were standing together that we understood his immediate problem and realized things had progressed much further than we had previously appreciated.

In the long-term care facility as he neared the end of his life, Jim was bedbound and eventually became unresponsive to Sadie and to the nursing staff. Nevertheless, one of our daughters has a vivid memory of coming to visit him during this time and calling out in a loud voice, "Hello, Uncle Jim!" She recalls that he reacted by sitting straight up in bed and looking directly at her. Although he did not say anything, Sadie and the nursing staff marveled at this unexpected response to a familiar voice.

We were greatly saddened when Jim died at the age of 70; Sadie's death followed four years later. In this example of dementia in our family, we see how the illness experience was compounded by Sadie's earlier and concurrent losses; by geographical distance between Sadie and her daughter, Donna; by Jim's inexorable decline; and by Sadie's valiant but unsuccessful efforts to cope with what was happening.

Donna and Chuck

After I retired from teaching, we relocated permanently to Florida where we have enjoyed many happy years. Even though our children and grandchildren live quite a distance from us, they visit frequently. They particularly enjoy our in-ground pool, so much so that our youngest grandchild once asked her mother if we could bring the pool with us when we next visited them. But some shadows came over our happiness in 2009 when some problems Donna was experiencing with short-term memory loss and occasional confusion led our geriatrician to refer her to a neurologist for a comprehensive evaluation. The result was a clinical diagnosis of mild cognitive impairment (MCI). We were told that dementia is not a part of normal aging and were comforted to learn that only about 15% of individuals with MCI go on to develop more serious forms of dementia or Alzheimer's disease. Still, this diagnosis was not completely benign and it signaled a change in both of our lives.

As we write this, Donna has short-term memory loss and some degree of confusion, although the latter seems to fluctuate on a daily or hourly basis. Her geriatrician recently described her as having mixed dementia with a particular focus on memory loss. Donna's problems typically are characterized by an inability to recall events that have just happened, people we have recently met, or things we have done lately. When we go out for lunch, choosing her meal from a lengthy menu sometimes seems challenging. In any local travels or during visits to our children's homes, Donna's confusion is often manifested by repeated questions about where we are going, where we are, or where we have been. Even though it is clear that such questions reflect a search for orientation and reassurance, it does not mean that the answers will be understood or recalled. That reality can be both annoying and frustrating to the person responding to such questions.

Typical questions when Donna wakes in the morning have to do with obligations she sometimes believes she may still have (Don't I have to go teach a class, give a presentation, or attend a meeting?); questions often have to do with where we are living (in Illinois? in St. Louis?), where our home is (Are we just visiting here?), and whose house this is (Jim and Sadie's?). Another set of questions relates to the whereabouts of Donna's father, mother, Uncle Jim, and Auntie Millie (her mother's youngest sister, with whom Donna and her mother were close). In fact, all of these people and everyone else in that generation of the family are now deceased and Donna is the oldest of her living cousins.

As we leave for home after dining out, Donna often asks repeatedly where her purse is, though she has not carried a purse since surgery on her shoulder more than three years ago. Other questions often concern the identities of people who are incorrectly thought to be visiting or who have visited us recently. It takes some practice and skill to follow the advice of our nurse practitioner daughter that the main goal in responding to such questions is not logic, but reassurance: "Everything is okay. Your purse is at home and I am taking care of everything else."

Despite these problems, Donna mostly retains her pleasant and outgoing personality. She talks in a genial way with me, as well as with friends and visitors. Granting that she may repeat statements or questions more than once in the course of a conversation, most people interact with Donna in an easy and friendly manner. Recently, during an evening spent with old friends and a few new people, Donna interacted with everyone in an amiable and easygoing style, though she may not have recognized all of the old acquaintances. The next morning she had no memory of that gathering. Similarly, a very caring cousin often talks with her by telephone about her daily activities; he is understanding when the conversation is interrupted by Donna's questions about how his parents are doing, as she does not recall that they have been dead for more than 15 years. Although Donna is handicapped by significant short-term memory loss and some degree of confusion, she otherwise continues to be socially adept in many ways. Nevertheless, some aspects of the companionship, sharing of daily trivia, and discussions of planned activities that are typical of individuals who have lived together for a long time are unavoidably impaired.

Like her grandmother Marie and many older adults with some degree of cognitive impairment or dementia, Donna's physical challenges are compounded by other health problems. She has what professionals call mild to moderate arthritis (although we view it as pretty severe); this led to the replacement of her left shoulder joint. Unfortunately, Donna's arthritis persists in her right shoulder and in both knees. She has, however, been told that she is not a good candidate for additional surgery, perhaps because she is somewhat frail and does not have the muscle strength she used to have. To assist with mobility, as well as getting up and down from a chair or in and out of a car, she wears a gait belt at all times and frequently uses a cane. A walker is a great help to stabilize her as she moves around our home and a wheelchair is very helpful during trips outside the house when she has to navigate longer distances, such as from the car to a restaurant or shopping mall. Life together generally moves more slowly now and many things take longer to carry out. Complaints of pain are intermittent, but usually seem to be treated adequately with acetaminophen.

Donna's complaints of dizziness or "feeling loopy" may be related to the combination of her cognitive impairment and arthritis. She also sleeps far more than she used to. We don't know the precise origin of her current sleeping pattern, but it is easier to cope with than other issues. Donna's own explanation attributes excessive sleeping to her multiple medicines, though her geriatrician and our nurse practitioner daughter disagree on that point. In addition, Donna often says that when she was younger and had to take tests in school, she would experience great anxiety and a "burning in her brain" that she now thinks may have resulted in wearing out some of her brain cells.

Not surprisingly, all of this means that many household chores have been shifted to me. I have learned to wash clothes reasonably well but I don't iron or sew. We are fortunate to have an arrangement with a very efficient and cheerful person who comes in at two-week intervals to clean the main living areas of our house. Because she often finds Donna still in bed when she arrives in the mid-morning, she calls Donna "the princess." We are equally blessed with sufficient resources to have trustworthy helpers do many chores around the house and yard that are now beyond either of our abilities.

My cooking skills are clearly limited, but frequent lunches at local eateries and an occasional evening meal at area restaurants often provide both nutritious food and leftovers for meals the next day. We have a very limited social life, and on the whole, live very quietly.

On two occasions, we were visited by a local deputy sheriff responding to Donna's telephone calls for assistance when she could not immediately locate me. (One time, I was trimming bushes out of sight in the front yard; the other time I was working quietly on the computer in the downstairs study.) In each case, the deputies were kind enough to appreciate our situation; they also reported that such calls were quite familiar to them. Now, we often link errands to a restaurant lunch and Donna is usually happy to wait in the car while I do what is needed. When she does not come along, we limit errands to short excursions, trying to undertake them during periods of daytime sleep for Donna. We talk together very clearly about the brief time that will be needed for such trips, and exchange our standard joke about promising not to call the sheriff's department (which Donna really no longer remembers doing). On rare occasions, perhaps once or twice a year when I must go out of town for a few days to attend a professional meeting, one of our daughters volunteers to stay with Donna for a week or so that overlaps my absence. We are both pleased to have that excuse to see them.

These days, it is common for our geriatrician, our children, and others to inquire both about Donna's health and well-being, and about what all of this means for me. Recently, our new Medicare Advantage insurance program sent a healthcare professional to visit our home to make similar inquiries. We are currently making arrangements with a home health agency that will provide a companion to stay with Donna when I need to be out of the house for a few hours.

Donna's health now apparently is as good as it can be. She is less interested and less able to be involved in activities like gardening or assembling puzzles that previously occupied much of her time, but she doesn't seem to miss such pursuits. She doesn't really engage in other activities that she used to enjoy like cleaning house, doing laundry, or preparing meals, although she still likes to wash dishes on some evenings.

For nearly nine years, Donna found great satisfaction in a stray cat that she took into our home and cared for devotedly. Sammie showed no interest in playing with toys, but he was always happy to sit on Donna's lap while she allowed her to brush his fur. He also liked sleeping next to her or on top of her. But recently, Donna came to the sad recognition that Sammie had to be euthanized because of some ongoing health problems that could not be corrected. Sammie's death has obviously been an important loss in Donna's life. In addition, what also is evident are Donna's ruminations and repetitive questions that have followed, such as: When and how did we get Sammie? Where is Sammie now? Is he dead? When or how did that happen? Why did we have to put him down? When will we get his ashes and what will we do with them? Donna always adds that Sammie was "a wonderful kitty" and that "she loved him very much."

Taking care of Donna and the household, while maintaining some level of professional activities involving research, writing, and editing, fills my days. Donna used to say that I was not really retired; my response was that I never wished to be retired if retirement meant giving up all of my academic and service interests. In any event, activities like fishing, boating, or golf under Florida's potentially harmful sun are not very appealing to fair-skinned people like me. I read avidly, mostly novels and historical works, along with publications relating to my academic interest in death, dying, and bereavement. The general attitude that has characterized my entire life is a pragmatic outlook that seeks to meet the challenges I encounter, as I confront them, as best I can.

Donna and I have both experienced losses in recent years. Those losses have involved challenges and called for efforts to cope with or face up to the trials that have come our way. But our attitude is that we just have to do whatever needs to be done. Clearly, Donna could not live alone; if I wasn't here, she would have to move in with one of our children (or have one of them move in with her). Alternatively, she would have to enter a long-term care facility, perhaps of the type in which our daughters work, one as a geriatric nurse practitioner, the other as a speech pathologist and manager of a rehabilitation department.

Some Lessons

- We have realized that dementia is insidious and often progressive; early signs are easily dismissed as inconsequential or petty eccentricities. But especially when they become more frequent, prominent, or persistent, such signs should be taken seriously and investigated appropriately. A complete medical examination should not be delayed by an understandable (though unhealthy) desire not to acknowledge what is happening.
- Although cognitive impairment in dementia typically is chronic, irreversible, and deepens over an extended period of time, that is not always the case. An individual's mental condition, like Donna's, may fluctuate in ways that are challenging for the person and those closest to her, but that also may offer opportunities to cherish many good times like those that are still part of our lives.
- Many people are unsure how to respond to encounters with dementia, as we were, but there now are numerous resources available (like this book and the *Living with Grief®* program, *The Longest Loss: Alzheimer's Disease and Dementia*, from Hospice Foundation of America) and organizations like the Alzheimer's Association that can provide guidance both to professionals and the public. We believe that failing to avail oneself of such resources

or focusing on keeping secrets only handicaps responses and complicates future prospects.

- Behavior, as we saw in the failed communication between Jim and us, can be an important means of communication when individuals are no longer able to express themselves verbally; being attentive to behavioral signs is imperative.

- Dementia can overwhelm family resources as it did in many ways in the case of both Marie and Jim; seeking assistance is neither improper nor inappropriate.

- Well-meaning family members, like Sadie, can exhaust themselves and endanger their own health while caring for a person with dementia. That is not helpful because a caregiver cannot be effective, especially over the long run, without caring for himself or herself.

- As we have seen in our family, how a person responds to a loved one with dementia often has much to do with that person's underlying personality and how he or she has coped with other challenges throughout life. Someone who has an anxious personality and has previously compensated by trying to control everything in life may not be willing to accept what is happening and may try to resist the loved one's decline, while another person who is more secure and more adaptable may adjust to the new and changing situation more easily and more readily.

- Some degree of relief or respite from the burdens of disease and caregiving can be helpful to both the person with dementia and family care providers; it is neither wrong nor selfish in these and other matters to seek "new normals" in life, to try to maintain interests outside the home, to arrange "time off," to rally informal and formal networks of support, and to make decisions about what is needed or wanted.

- When families can no longer cope on their own with the burdens associated with advanced dementia (as became evident in the situations of Marie and Jim), there is no disgrace in seeking assistance from professionals in home care, long-term care facilities, specialized memory units, and hospice programs.

- Transitions in care, such as those that occurred when Jim was admitted first to a hospital and then to a long-term care facility, can involve difficult decisions and changes for both the individual and for family members, and sometimes leads to disagreements among them; such transitions need to be based on established goals of care and careful discussion by all involved.

- Individuals with dementia who are, or appear to be, unresponsive to others in their surroundings should be treated with respect and dignity; continuing to talk to and with them (as our daughter did with Jim), to offer companionship (the "gift of presence"), and to provide appropriate forms of stimulation, is highly desirable.
- Individuals with any form of dementia, at whatever stage, remain persons who should be loved and appreciated for who they are, not what they can or cannot do; they deserve care and assistance from family members, friends, volunteer and professional care providers, and their communities.
- Although our family has not experienced what some have interpreted as rejection by individuals with dementia of spouses or other previously-close relatives, it should not be surprising that individuals with advanced dementia might reach out for new relationships when they can no longer recognize family members, find current surroundings strange or scary, or simply seek companionship and some degree of happiness.
- In situations involving Alzheimer's disease, other forms of dementia, and cognitive impairment in general, appreciating the likelihood of grief reactions to losses of all types throughout the course of the disease and afterwards can facilitate better coping and a greater willingness to seek out appropriate forms of assistance. Our own such losses independent of the disease include the death of Sadie's first husband, Tony, and of our cat, Sammie. Individuals will inevitably pursue their own grief journeys, but they can often be helped by dementia support groups, hospice bereavement programs, or other forms of grief support.
- Late-stage dementia or Alzheimer's disease, as experienced by Marie and Jim, can have broad repercussions in family relationships, financial, legal, and other dimensions; whenever possible, it helps families to address some of these matters when the individual with the disease is still competent to participate in decision-making. Jim did this well in advance of his decline by settling personal and financial matters and by completing advance directives about health care.

Donna and I hope that this description of encounters with dementia in our family and the lessons that emerge from these experiences will be of help to others in similar situations.

Donna M. Corr, RN, MS in Nursing, took early retirement from her position as Professor in the Nursing Faculty of St. Louis Community College at Forest Park, St. Louis, Missouri. Her publications include Hospice Care: Principles and Practice *(Springer, 1983),* Hospice Approaches to Pediatric Care *(Springer, 1985),* Nursing Care in an Aging Society *(Springer, 1990),* Sudden Infant Death Syndrome: Who Can Help and How *(Springer, 1991), and* Handbook of Childhood Death and Bereavement *(Springer, 1996), all co-edited with Charles Corr, as well as two dozen book chapters and articles in professional journals.*

Charles A. Corr, PhD, is a member of: the Board of Directors, Suncoast Hospice Institute, an affiliate of Empath Health in Clearwater, Florida; the International Work Group on Death, Dying, and Bereavement; the Association for Death Education and Counseling; and the ChiPPS (Children's Project on Palliative/Hospice Services) E-Journal Work Group of the National Hospice and Palliative Care Organization. A frequent contributor to Hospice Foundation of America's Journeys: A Newsletter to Help in Bereavement, *Dr. Corr's publications include more than three dozen books and booklets, along with over 100 chapters and articles in professional journals. His most recent book, co-authored with Donna Corr, is the seventh edition of* Death & Dying, Life & Living *(Wadsworth, 2013).*

CHAPTER 5

Birds sing after a storm: When Dementia Caregiving Ends

Jennifer Elison and Chris McGonigle

"Birds sing after a storm; why shouldn't people feel as free to delight in whatever sunlight remains to them?" (Rose Kennedy, 1974)

In our book *Liberating Losses* (Elison & McGonigle, 2003), we focused on relief following a death, a subject the literature had addressed only fleetingly, if at all. Although our research was anecdotal and personal rather than quantitative and academic, we had hoped to reassure the grieving public that positive emotions were perfectly acceptable following a death. We also hoped that such reassurance would lead to more widespread public acceptance of such outcomes. However, 11 years on, we have been surprised and discouraged to find that, with a few exceptions, this has not been the case, and the bereaved still labor under many myths and misconceptions about the grief process.

Each of us had experienced a "liberating loss." Jennifer's young husband had been emotionally abusive. The day after she asked him for a divorce, he was killed in a car accident. She grappled with an intense and contradictory array of emotions, but the foremost was relief at being free from an abusive marriage, and that her troubled spouse had finally found peace.

Chris's experience was quite different. Her beloved husband Don was diagnosed with multiple sclerosis at the age of 33, and suffered an agonizing downhill course until he died at age 46 in a nursing home. At the time of Don's diagnosis, her daughter was 4 years old and her son just 18 months; she had to console them throughout his decline and death as well. She had mourned each loss of mobility and Don's slow withdrawal from family life, and felt relieved when his suffering was finally over.

Both of us experienced non-traditional, or disenfranchised, emotions after our husbands died, Jennifer to a greater degree, Chris somewhat less. (The term *disenfranchised grief* was coined by Kenneth Doka in 1989 and refers to losses that are not openly acknowledged, socially sanctioned, or publicly mourned.) Perhaps because researchers feared alienating subjects, grief inventories rarely asked, "What don't you miss about this person or situation?" and disenfranchised grievers had consequently been largely overlooked in the literature. Those who don't seem to be grieving "properly," that is, according to cultural norms, are denounced as frivolous, shallow, or unnatural. Our subjects would have identified with some of the widows who had lost husbands in the 9/11 attacks on the World Trade Center. These women were revered until they began remarrying and reclaiming their own identities. Then their devotion to their late husbands was questioned, and some were accused of rushing to replace their dead mates.

We gathered many similar stories from other disenfranchised grievers for our book, and were often surprised when people who had heard of our project approached us asking, sometimes pleadingly, to tell their stories, on the condition that their names be changed. Truly, we felt, we had tapped into a societal taboo. Some of our subjects, like Jennifer, had been in abusive relationships. Others' family members or spouses were mentally ill; they never knew when a distress call would come in the middle of the night. One woman eloquently summed up the complexity of her post-death feelings: "I'm sure you understand that when I talk about relief, it doesn't mean I don't wish he were alive. I'd give anything to have John alive" (Elison & McGonigle, 2003, p. 66). The secrecy these grievers were forced to maintain made their already shameful feelings more difficult to process. All our subjects found themselves victims of societal expectations as they tried to hide their relief—which some went so far as to call joy and elation—and newfound sense of freedom. Most were able to share their feelings with a trusted friend or family member, but some were completely alone.

Analyzing our interview material, we proposed three types of post-death relief (our subjects had lost spouses, parents, or children at various ages, including newborns, to illnesses brief and prolonged, as well as suicide). The first was *altruistic relief*, which followed when the dead person had suffered a great deal. *Dual relief*, our second category, resulted in positive feelings because the survivor was relieved for him or herself as well. *Relationship relief*, our third category, followed a very emotionally difficult or abusive relationship.

After the publication of *Liberating Losses*, Jennifer was reminded once again of how risky it is to speak publicly of relief. In January 2007, *Newsweek* magazine published her "My Turn" essay, "The Stage of Grief No One Admits To: Relief." The piece struck a nerve with the public, generating an unusually large reader response. Many readers wrote to thank her for her honesty and to tell her that their own losses felt very liberating. This woman's letter is typical: "Both of my parents passed away last year and I felt no grief, only relief, because of some of the reasons you outlined in the article. I am not ashamed of these feelings." However, Jennifer also heard, in tones loud and clear, from those with differing views. In the *Newsweek* response chat box, via snail mail and in phone calls, readers denounced her as callous, cold, and unfeeling, and questioned her credentials as a therapist and a human being.

This distrust and vilification of positive post-bereavement feelings has a special relevance to American culture in light of the huge increase in those suffering from Alzheimer's disease and related dementias (ADRD). Currently, one in three senior citizens in the United States dies from ADRD. This enormous number will take an exponential toll on survivors, since, in 2013, approximately 15.4 million caregivers volunteered about 17 billion hours of care; most of these caregivers are family members (Alzheimer's Association, 2014). The news only gets worse. According to recent projections, Chris's home state of Montana will see a 50% increase in ADRD between 2014 and 2025; so will Jennifer's home state of Florida (AARP, 2014). A hospice nurse we interviewed for *Liberating Losses* told us, "...I do think, more than any other kind of death, that family members of people with Alzheimer's experience massive relief" (2003, p. 53).

The stresses experienced by family members caring for those with ADRD have been well-documented in the literature. A grief-stress model of ADRD caregiving was proposed by Noyes and colleagues in 2010. The model identified the primary stressors as *relational deprivation* (losses of companionship, communication, support, changes in the dynamic of the relationship, and hope for improvement) and *role overload* (losses of personal freedom, opportunities for socialization, work, and recreation, and personal health and identity). The caregivers reported feeling loneliness, regret, hopelessness, confusion, and agitation, as well as stress related to burden, social/work life constriction, and role captivity (Noyes et al., 2010).

The burden is heavy indeed for this invisible army, mostly made up of middle-aged women who may also be raising children, holding down jobs, and tending their own households. By its nature, dementia will deprive caregiving of one of its chief pleasures, that of recognition and appreciation from the loved one. One study called the ADRD experience "dual dying": survivors are forced to witness two deaths because the personality vanishes long before the body gives out (Jones & Martinson, 1992). The combination of hopelessness, grinding physical work, financial worries, forced withdrawal from previous supportive friendships and affiliations, and grief as a loved one dies of this diabolical illness will seem overwhelming at times.

Certainly ADRD caregivers deserve the feelings of relief and freedom that follow such a protracted and consuming experience, but the bereavement culture has yet to catch up. Journalist Ruth Davis Konigsberg notes that "Our grief culture maintains that 'everyone's grief is unique,' and then offers a uniform set of instructions" (2011, p. 15). In particular, the persistence of stage models is, according to Konigsberg, "the idea that won't die" (2011, p. 1). We goal-oriented, deterministic Americans have little patience with the obstreperous and unpredictable life experience we know as grieving. We want to organize it, tame it, then "power through it" step-by-step, checking each one off as we go. Some guides even suggest a timetable of as little as three months to get through them all. Elisabeth Kübler-Ross's Five Stage Model had an undeniable appeal; "If we had seven fingers we would have had seven stages," joked a colleague. While we owe Kübler-Ross a debt of gratitude for taking grief out of the closet and putting it on the coffee table, her stage-model theory has become a stumbling block for many who feel they don't fit the mold. Dr. Richard Schulz, Distinguished Service Professor of Psychiatry, Director of the University of Pittsburgh's Center for Social and Urban Research, and the author of numerous studies on the effects of illness on patients and family members, describes the Kübler-Ross model in the following way: "It's a nice story, it's believable, but it's not true" (R. Schulz, personal communication, September 18, 2014).

"Whether it is death and dying, successful sex, coping with life's many stresses, or baking zucchini bread—it seems that what we all want is a recipe, a neat package of stages or skills that says this is how it is. With the exception of zucchini bread, this does not seem to be the case," wrote Wasow and Coons (1988, p.27). Although this quip was written over 25 years ago, a recent online search for self-help bereavement books (6,662 titles) reveals that Americans are still searching for the perfect map for bereavement. Many of the titles such as *Tear Soup: A Recipe for Healing After Loss* (Schweibert & DeKlyen, 2005); *Healing After Loss: Daily Meditations for Working Through Grief* (Hickman, 1994); and *On Grief and Grieving: Finding the Meaning of Grief Through the Five Stages of Loss* (Kübler-Ross, Kessler, & Shriver, 2014), lead the public to believe that bereavement involves a prescriptive, step-by-step process. Entering "bereavement workbooks" in the search category at Amazon.com results in no fewer than 126 titles, reinforcing the idea that by following the suggestions in a formulated process, one's grief will be effectively alleviated.

The digital age allows anyone and everyone to post comments and videos proclaiming the latest and greatest solutions to personal problems. YouTube has over 120 videos that offer help and guidance during bereavement. While these videos are well-intentioned, the viewer would do well to remember that anyone at all, credentialed or not, can post on this site. Even authoritative web sites such as WebMD and PsychCentral still advocate a five-stage model, with the latter declaring that stages are "universal."

Yet in a number of significant ways, ADRD is changing the face of bereavement. Jones and Martinson (1992) interviewed 13 men and women who provided care to their spouses or parents with Alzheimer's disease with the length of time of caregiving ranging from 3 to 10 years. Most (85%) were interviewed within 12 months of the death.

Fifty-four percent of the sample indicated that the period of most intense grief was during the caregiving period. Part of the grief was connected to either saying a final goodbye or the inability to communicate a proper goodbye with the loved one. "I couldn't cry much afterwards. I'd cried my heart out before," one daughter reported (Jones & Martinson, 1992, p. 173). In Hospice Foundation of America's book *Living With Grief: Alzheimer's Disease,* Meuser, Marwit, and Sanders stated that caregiver grief is "relatively indistinguishable from post-death grief in personal impact and meaning" (2004, p.175). Noyes and colleagues added to this finding, noting that while previous researchers had called this "anticipatory grief," researchers are beginning to recognize that caregiver grieving is in fact "true grief," and is at least as stressful as that experienced post-death (Noyes et al., 2010). The up-and-down nature of ADRD caregiving, in which the person receiving care can seem perfectly lucid and appropriate one day and devastatingly absent the next, makes the caregiver experience particularly challenging. Additionally, what has often been identified as depression has been properly reclassified as grief, and caregivers do plenty of it before the death of their loved one with ADRD.

"After what seemed like a 10-year funeral, many caregivers felt ready for their family members to be taken from them completely," Jones and Martinson observed (1992, p. 174). Their study is the only one we found that attempted to describe types of relief. They claimed that *sorrowful relief* was felt by those whose relief was mingled with sorrow and grief. Typically, those who described this pattern of relief were providing care to family members who were still able to respond with recognition and affection. For some, *sorrowful relief* was associated with difficulty in letting go of painful memories of the disease process itself. The second pattern of relief, *guilty relief*, was defined as relief associated with guilt related to a variety of sources. For example, some participants acknowledged feeling guilty for experiencing the emotion of relief. Some indicated that the guilt feelings were associated with difficult decisions, i.e., institutionalization, made during the illness. The final pattern of relief, *grateful relief*, was experienced by those caregivers whose loved ones had lost their ability to communicate in a meaningful manner. They had also experienced anticipatory grieving, and felt comfortable with the care they had given. Seventy-seven percent of the sample described relief associated with their bereavement. The authors remind us that to experience relief does not mean that no sorrow was associated with the death. Instead, the relief was a component of the grieving process (Jones & Martinson, 1992).

Schulz, Newsom, Fleissner, Decamp, and Nieboer conducted a review of 17 studies related to bereavement following family caregiving. Their findings support the idea that relatives had few difficulties adjusting to the death of their family members. Although they found some short-term negative outcomes associated with the death, they found evidence for positive outcomes for the care provider such as relief from the burden of care and improved well-being. They speculated that the relief may have been attributed to an ending of the patient's suffering as well (1997).

A quantitative study conducted by Schulz et al. (2003) and appearing in the *New England Journal of Medicine* confirmed Jones and Martinson's findings that feelings of relief are common among family caregivers of persons with ADRD. The 217 individuals studied were participants in the Resources for Enhancing Alzheimer's Caregiver Health (REACH) investigation that included six geographic locations. In this longitudinal study, participants were assessed at baseline; at 6, 12, and 18 months; and following the death of the family member. The researchers collected data on the amount of assistance the family member gave to the patient, the amount of burden felt by the family member (as measured by the Revised Memory and Behavior Problems Checklist), and depressive symptoms of the family member, as well as medication use. Following the death of the family member from dementia, data was collected to assess a variety of factors, including amount of time the patient felt pain prior to death, relief felt by the caregiver, the extent relief may have been experienced by the patient, and bereavement support group utilization.

Schulz and his colleagues found that caregiving family members exhibited unexpected resilience in their adaptation to the death and that their levels of depression decreased to pre-caregiving levels within one year following the death. Additionally, only about 25% of the participants reported feelings of depression a year after the death, with few feeling the need to participate in bereavement-related services. Interviewed about his findings, Schulz pointed out a distinct difference between the experience of those who had placed a loved one in a nursing home and those who had cared for him or her at home. "You don't get this closure when you put someone in a long-term care facility," he said. "You don't get the release that people who have experienced the death of a loved one do" (Associated Press, 2013). Most germane to our subject, however, is the finding that 72% of the caregivers indicated that they felt "somewhat" or "very much" relieved by the death of the patient. Even more impressive, 90% believed it was a relief to the patient (Schulz et al., 2003).

Although the media usually ignores such studies, this one made national news: "Caregivers Often Feel Relief After Alzheimer's Death," announced the Associated Press. One of the major television networks also featured the study on its evening broadcast. The real news here, however, is that this study made the news, when relief following such grueling caregiving seems so natural a reaction.

Haley, Bergman, Roth, McVie, and Gaugler (2008) reported that the death of a care recipient with Alzheimer's led to a decrease in symptoms of depression in the caregiver. The study included 254 spouses of persons for whom care had been provided at home and who died from AD. Subjects were part of the NYU Caregiver Intervention (NYUCI) Study. Baseline data was collected and the subjects were then randomly assigned to either an enhanced group for support and counseling or a control condition. Data collection continued every 4 months with the same instrument used at baseline. Additionally, assessments were completed every 6 months during the first year and, if available, until the death of the care recipient. At least one, and sometimes two, interviews were conducted either by telephone or face-to-face following the death of the care recipient.

The results of this longitudinal study suggested that, in both the treatment and the control groups, supportive caregiver attention and care while the patient was alive helped alleviate post-bereavement depressive symptoms. Further, as in the Schulz study, the decrease in depressive symptoms was most pronounced in spouses who had not placed their husbands or wives in nursing homes. The authors theorized that supportive intervention may alleviate depression after the death of the spouse (Haley et al., 2008).

Similarly, Chan, Livingston, Jones, and Sampson conducted a meta-analysis of 31 studies and found that relief was an outcome for many caregivers. "Carer relief after death is common and related to positive experiences, less burden and acknowledged grief in the caring period, as well as consistent support before and after death" (2013, p. 14). The relief felt by the survivors also was associated with feeling that the death was a relief for the individual with ADRD (Chan et al., 2013).

A study by Jessica Allen, a student of Haley, links relief and resilience even more closely. While only 8% of her sample had a primary diagnosis of dementia, Allen found that a lack of relief could lead to negative outcomes. Her doctoral dissertation, published in 2012, was based on her study of 61 caregiver-spouses whose husbands and wives had been enrolled in one of two hospice programs in the Southeast. Interviews took place approximately 11 months after the death of the care recipient. Relief was especially likely when the caregiver perceived that there had been a great degree of emotional suffering on the part of the care recipient (Allen, 2012).

This body of research, which removes any doubt of the existence of positive post-bereavement feelings in ADRD survivors, could provide hope and a sense of normalcy for other relieved grievers. The difficulty lies in bridging the gap between scholarly writing and the social norms that guide the lives of everyday people. For most, old beliefs still prevail, and the concepts of relief and resilience have yet to find recognition and approval.

George Bonanno, whose research on loss and survivors of trauma spans decades, speculates in his book *The Other Side of Sadness* (2009) on the possible reasons for this disconnect. He theorizes that Western countries expect bereavement to be difficult and painful; therefore we assume that sadness and grief will be constant companions for the bereaved. And because we care about the feelings of others and pay attention to those feelings, we tend to be astonished when someone does not react with pain and sorrow. Bonanno explains that relief and positive feelings can seem contradictory to the grieving process. "There is something counterintuitive about putting positive emotions and grief in the same sentence. Historically, positive emotions received almost no attention in the bereavement literature and when they were mentioned it was almost always in the context of denial. It was assumed that a joyous emotion during grieving could only interfere with or suppress the normal process of working through the loss" (2009, p. 36). His observations are especially relevant to the bereavement experience following ADRD deaths.

Trying to fit into an outdated stage model, or have well-meaning grief counselors try to make the model fit, has never worked very well, but it may be particularly maladaptive for ADRD survivors. They have witnessed a wrenching series of declines and have already done most of their grieving; they may have no need for "working through their grief." Most of these grievers are middle-aged themselves and, if their bodies haven't already informed them of the fact, the loss of a parent or spouse surely has reminded them that life is short. If grief counselors or social workers are still trying to apply an outdated stage model, encouraging visible signs of grief as evidence that they are "processing" their grief, and discouraging new relationships or plans of action in the belief that big decisions should be put off for at least a year, they may be doing these survivors a disservice. If these professionals truly believe that everyone's grief is unique, they must be willing to accept that this cohort may be ready, even eager, to move forward and should encourage them in that endeavor. While these grievers may not know exactly how to move forward with their lives, the idea of reinventing themselves in their new roles deserves respect and careful nurturing.

Unfortunately, this notion has been slow to catch on. In August, 2010, Jennifer attended a two-day workshop in Portland, Oregon sponsored by the End-of-Life Nursing Education Consortium (ELNEC). The ELNEC project was founded in 2000 to provide education to nurses to improve palliative care. Participants receive ELNEC certification upon completion of the seminar with the intent that they will share their knowledge with other nurses. The ELNEC speakers were all experts in the fields of palliative and hospice care as well as bereavement services. Evidence-based materials were presented on such topics as pain management, spirituality, communicating with the dying, alleviating physical symptoms that accompany the dying process, and bereavement care. The discussions were robust and the content was pertinent and timely. The Kübler-Ross model was not held up as the quintessential road map for grieving and the speakers acknowledged that humans are unique in their experience of bereavement. However, Jennifer was struck by the fact that relief was not mentioned as a component of the bereavement process, and disappointed that presenters had missed an opportunity for sharing valuable information.

She was disappointed as well when she read a study by Holman, Perisho, Edwards, and Mlakar (2010) called *The Myths of Coping with Loss in Undergraduate Psychiatric Nursing Books*. The authors examined how myths of coping with loss are perpetuated in undergraduate textbooks used in mental health and psychiatric nursing courses. They compared 23 undergraduate psychiatric nursing texts published between 1998 and 2009 for how many of these texts contained outdated information about grieving (for example, that there are predictable stages to grief, emotions need to be processed, lack of expression of negative emotions equates to pathology) rather than evidence-based findings (people grieve in a variety of ways, lack of obvious grief does not necessarily mean pathology, repressive coping is perfectly healthy for some).

The authors' findings are disheartening. Eighty-seven percent of the textbooks restated myths relating to stages or predictable patterns of grief. The majority (69.6%) advised students that negative emotions cannot be prevented and 65.2% of the books contained information telling nurses that a lack of expression of negative emotions is indicative of pathology. Just as discouraging was the lack of evidence-based findings. None of the textbooks included any mention of resilience, positive growth, or any positive emotions associated with loss. The authors lament that, "Despite this multidisciplinary body of research questioning stage theories of grief, these theories continue to be used in end-of-life care and are widely disseminated to healthcare professionals" (Holman et al., 2010, p. 487).

Curious now, Jennifer decided to conduct an informal poll of 25 students in a fall 2014 research class she was teaching. The students were all experienced nurses, with 3 to 20 years in practice. Borrowing a question from the Holman study, she asked, "Do you expect to see bereaved families responding in a predictable way?" The majority (64%) said yes. Some of the students specifically referred to the Kübler-Ross stage theory. When asked to elaborate about what assumptions the nurses would make if the person did not appear distressed by the loss, most replied that the person must be "in denial." As the Institute of Medicine noted in its yearly report, *Dying in America*, "recent knowledge gains have not necessarily translated to improved patient care" (2014, para. 11).

Hospice and palliative care professionals must recognize the fact that, with the Alzheimer's epidemic ravaging our aging population, bereavement care must be offered during the caregiving phase, because this is when the most painful grieving occurs—not, for most, after a death. As Haley (2008) discovered, caregiver intervention appears to be very useful in easing post-bereavement depression, since family caregivers can be helped to cope with their grief and assisted in making difficult decisions regarding the care of their loved one. Both Schulz et al. (2003) and Haley et al. (2008) found that nursing home placement does not result in the same positive emotions as those that followed a death; it simply shifts the caregiver's responsibilities down the street or across town. Healthcare workers need to be aware of these findings and remember that helping caregivers care for family members at home, if that is their wish, results in less guilt post-death and a greater sense of well-being after a year. When appropriate, healthcare workers can reassure caregivers that their ordeal will not last forever, and that they can expect to feel, and be entitled to feel, relief and satisfaction after their loved one dies.

We do not mean to suggest that these survivors will not have work to do reclaiming an identity that has been submerged by years of caregiving, but we wish to distinguish this work of self-rediscovery, which has the potential to be joy-filled, from "grief work." We hope that healthcare workers can remind caregivers that their sacrifices made a difference and enable them to look toward the future with renewed zest.

Jennifer Elison, EdD, is an associate professor of nursing at the University of Great Falls and incorporates end-of-life and bereavement content across the curriculum. She is an advanced practice registered nurse and licensed therapist and has counseled bereaved individuals and families in transition. She founded the Helena Life Transition Network and served as the board president. Dr. Elison provided counseling services to clients enrolled in the Advanced Illness Coordinated Care program sponsored by Blue Cross and Blue Shield of Montana. She is the co-author of Liberating Losses: When Death Brings Relief *(Perseus, 2003).*

Chris McGonigle, PhD, is a freelance writer whose work has appeared in Woman's World, Woman's Day, Family Circle, Good Housekeeping, *and other national magazines. She is the author of* Surviving Your Spouse's Chronic Illness: A Compassionate Guide *(Henry Holt, 1999) and the co-author of* Liberating Losses: When Death Brings Relief *(Perseus, 2003). She has served as adjunct professor of English at a number of Montana colleges and universities.*

REFERENCES

AARP. (2014). *AARP Bulletin/Real Possibilities.* October 2014, p. 34.

Allen, J. (2012). *Bereavement outcomes among spousal hospice caregivers: The role of rumination, feelings of relief, and perceived suffering* (Doctoral dissertation). Retrieved from http://scholarcommons.usf.edu/cgi/viewcontent.cgi?article=54x

Alzheimer's Association (2014). *Alzheimer's Disease Facts and Figures.* Retrieved from http://www.alz.org/downloads/facts_figures_2014.pdf

Associated Press. (2003). *Study: Caregivers Often Feel Relief After Alzheimer's Death.* Retrieved from http://www.nbcnews.com/id/3475868/ns/health-alzheimer's_disease

Bonanno, G. (2009). *The other side of sadness: What the new science of bereavement tells us about life after loss.* New York, NY: Basic Books.

Chan, D., Livingston, G., Jones, L., & Sampson, E. L. (2013). Grief reactions in dementia carers: A systematic review. *International Journal of Geriatric Psychiatry, 28,* 1-17.

Doka, K. J. (Ed.) (1989). *Disenfranchised grief: Recognizing hidden sorrow.* Lexington, MA: Lexington Books.

Elison, J., & McGonigle, C. (2003). *Liberating losses: When death brings relief.* Cambridge, MA: Perseus Books.

Haley, W., Bergman, E., Roth, D., McVie, T., & Gaugler, J. (2008). Long-term effects of bereavement and caregiver intervention on dementia caregiver depressive symptoms. *The Gerontologist, 48*(6), 732-740.

Holman, E. A., Perisho, J., Edwards, A., & Mlakar, N. (2010). The myths of coping with loss in undergraduate psychiatric nursing books. *Research in Nursing and Health, 33*, 486-499.

Institute of Medicine. (2014). *Dying in America: Improving quality and honoring individual preferences near the end of life (brief report).* Retrieved from http://www.iom.edu/~/media/Files/Report%20 Files/2014/EOL/Report%20Brief.pdf

Jones, P., & Martinson, I. (1992). The experience of bereavement in caregivers of family members with Alzheimer's disease. *IMAGE: Journal of Nursing Scholarship, 24*(3), 172-176.

Konigsberg, R. (2011). *The truth about grief.* New York, NY: Simon & Schuster.

Meuser, T., Marwit, S., & Sanders, S. (2004). Assessing grief in family caregivers. In K. J. Doka (Ed.), *Living with grief: Alzheimer's disease* (pp. 169-198). Washington, DC: Hospice Foundation of America.

Noyes, B., Hill, R., Hicken, B., Luptak, M., Rupper, R., Dailey, N., & Bair, B. (2010). Review: The role of grief in dementia caregiving. *American Journal of Alzheimer's Disease and Other Dementias, 25*, 9-17. doi: 10.1177/1533317509333902

Schulz, R., Newsom, J., Fleissner, K., Decamp, A., & Nieboer, A. (1997). The effects of bereavement after family caregiving. *Aging & Mental Health, 1*(3), 269-282.

Schulz, R., Mendelsohn, A., Haley, W., Mahoney, D., Allen, R., Zhang, S., Thompson, L., & Belle, S. (2003). End-of-life care and the effects of bereavement on family caregivers of persons with dementia. *New England Journal of Medicine, 349,* 1936-1942.

Wasow, M., & Coons, D. (1988). Widows and widowers of Alzheimer's victims. *Journal of Independent Social Work, 2*(2), 21-32. doi: 10.1300/J283v02n02_03

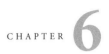

Voices:
An Unexpected Loss

Cris Abrams

I've often thought of my mom in the many years since she died from Alzheimer's disease. My experience as her caregiver was probably similar to that of many others in such circumstances. But I hope that my story might help others avoid a loss that I did not expect.

My family's journey through dementia officially started in the neurologist's office, although we suspected something was wrong months earlier. My mother had been given a series of tests and I was there to hear the results. The doctor said Mom was in the early stage of Alzheimer's and that it would be better for her not to be living alone.

My mother and I had always been close. I know some mother-daughter relationships are difficult; they can be tense and distant, but not ours. For example, when my father died 15 years earlier, Mom and I went to Europe on a trip she and Dad had planned for themselves. We had a great time and our relationship continued to grow over the years. More recently, I had been taking care of her long distance. I would drive three hours every three or four weeks to check up on her and make sure all was well.

My older brother and his family also lived a couple of hours away from Mom, but in another direction. He would call her but rarely visit. He checked in on her occasionally but wasn't overly concerned, probably because I was over there regularly. I started visiting a little more often because I was noticing a gradual decline and signs of dementia, though we didn't have a name for it at that time. She was putting tags on things like the kitchen timer with instructions on how to set it, and placing little notes around the place to remind herself of different things. We were coping; I was there, I was on top of it, I knew that this was going on and I didn't think that she was in danger at that time. Because my brother didn't see her as often, when he did eventually visit, it was kind of shocking to him and he said that something has to be done, that we have to fix this right away. I was used to seeing her and he wasn't, which turned out to be a good thing because he convinced me to get her checked out by a doctor.

So, after the neurologist discussed the test results and confirmed our suspicions, I called my brother and we agreed that Mom should live in an assisted living facility. She was still capable of taking care of herself for the most part, but needed others to make sure she was alright. I thought she could stay where she was a little while longer but my brother thought we should act immediately. We agreed that we each would start looking but I was surprised when my brother called only a couple of weeks later to say he had found Mom a place in an assisted living facility near him. I protested that I hadn't completed my research, but he was insistent, saying that we may lose the opportunity, so I gave in.

I found the sudden shift in my brother's interest in Mom to be very jarring. He went from almost total lack of involvement to, "We have to do this *now*. I am going to do this." I had always been the one Mom and Dad relied on. In all honesty, it made me proud that they had that kind of respect for me. Then, all of a sudden, I felt like that was ripped out of my hands. I had been looking after Mom for years, but in a matter of only a few weeks, she would be gone to the assisted living facility and my brother would be taking over. He assured me we would discuss all decisions that had to be made, but I was sad that Mom would not be living nearby.

The facility near my brother was very nice, and less expensive than any I could have found where I live. Mom had a bedroom, living room, small kitchen, and full bathroom. She was able to bring her own furniture, so was surrounded by familiar things. My brother and his wife added some cheery wallpaper. Things were off to a good start. My brother took over paying Mom's bills. He stopped by weekly and brought her to his home for Sunday dinner; she enjoyed his attention. I was happy to see my brother taking good care of Mom, allaying my fears, which I realized were probably more about my not taking care of Mom anymore.

I visited every couple of months, staying in her little apartment so we could enjoy ourselves, together. I noticed Mom was developing ways to cope with her memory loss. For instance, she would tune the TV in the living room to one channel and the TV in her bedroom to another, so when she wanted to "change" the channel, she would just go to the other room. I also noticed other changes. She stopped reading because, she said, she wanted to save her eyes, but I believe she couldn't understand the words anymore. And, although the facility took people to the mall, she wouldn't go because she was afraid she would get lost.

During this time, I got married and did something I had always wanted to do. I wore Mom's wedding dress. She was so happy that day and was so proud to see me in her dress. My wedding was small and informal; I think my brother wanted to give me away, but I was in my 30s when I married and saw no need for that kind of formality. I think that hurt him, but we never talked about it.

Mom continued to live in her apartment for several years, and I continued to visit every couple of months. I always told my brother when I was coming to town; he always was invited to come out to dinner with us or I'd take Mom over to his house to visit. We were close. Although Mom's memory continued to decline, she still recognized everyone, could communicate well, and was able to be relatively independent.

Unfortunately, a cold developed into something more severe and Mom was hospitalized. I was horrified to see her tied to the bed and in adult diapers. I was told that was necessary because staff could not always be available to take her to the bathroom; she was secured to the bed because she had Alzheimer's and they didn't want her to wander. It made me very sad to see my strong, independent mother subjected to this. But it was obvious that Mom needed more care than the assisted living facility could provide. Her options were either a nursing home or moving in with one of us. My brother stepped up and said she could live with him. I had confidence in him. He had been doing a great job taking care of Mom, going to see her, taking her to his house for visits. There was no doubt in my mind, I had no reservation.

My brother, his wife, and their grown son and daughter lived in a three-bedroom home. My nephew gave up his bedroom for Mom.

At this point, her dementia was worsening. She was much less accepting, more easily agitated, even paranoid at times, so they were having to cope with that. Mom's memory was getting worse and she had to be reminded to do basic things like comb her hair. Sometimes she would forget to eat or forget that she had eaten. She also needed help getting dressed. To a large extent, she needed to be told what to do and when to do it. She could no longer fully understand what was going on around her. Fortunately, she knew when she had to go to the bathroom.

I think they expected Mom to act like an adult. My sister-in-law thought Mom should be more appreciative. My nephew began calling her "my crazy grandmother." Though disrespectful, I don't think it was malicious. But they clearly didn't understand the disease and that she was no longer the person everybody knew. She needed help doing things, and they didn't seem to understand that wasn't her fault. They would share their observations with me, that things weren't right and they didn't understand why she did this or that, and I thought, yes, that's the disease, that's the way it happens. I just nodded. I might have reacted differently had I known what was going to happen down the road.

I often stayed with Mom so my brother's family could go away for the day or the weekend. I sometimes took Mom away and we stayed in a hotel. On one getaway, we went to where her parents had spent the winter when she was eight years old. Even with Alzheimer's, she understood that she was visiting a place she had been as a child. We talked about it all the way there and she described landmarks she remembered. We actually may have found the cement gateway to the neighborhood where she had stayed. At least, she thought she did, and it made her happy. These getaways were not easy for me because of the possibility Mom would wander, and I got little sleep. Mom, however, seemed to enjoy these outings and I was happy to give her some pleasure.

She had been living with my brother and his family for maybe three or four months when he called and said that she had to go to a nursing home. I didn't believe Mom was quite at that point yet. Though she needed assistance, I believed she could still live a fairly normal life. My husband and I talked it over and agreed she should come stay with us. My brother was fine with that; actually, I believe he was relieved. I think, in retrospect, there were pressures building up at home; his wife was feeling unappreciated, it was crowded, and I think he probably had had enough.

I was back to being Mom's main caregiver, a role I had relinquished some time ago. I was happy she was at my house. From my perspective,

I work, have a husband, take care of my Mom, take care of *me*; but I realize that I'm also having to cope with changes beyond those I see in Mom. I have less time for other things; we now have someone in our house during the day for Mom; our nighttime is limited because we can no longer simply jump up and go out to dinner because we have to think about Mom.

Occasionally, we got a break when my brother stayed with Mom in my home, returning the favor as I had done for him so many times in his home.

I was happy that I could care for Mom and keep her from having to go into a facility at that point. I was grateful that my husband was so willing to participate, because you need that support. I knew that at some point she would have to go into a facility but I just wanted to delay that as long as I could.

Sometimes, taking care of Mom was challenging. One chilly January morning she was quite upset because she thought I had moved us to a much colder part of the country. Another time, she woke up in the middle of the night, all excited that her mother (who had died long before) was coming for a visit and wanted to make sure I had room for her to stay. Sometimes caring for Mom was just plain stressful. She might suddenly refuse to do something for no logical reason; the Alzheimer's made it difficult for her to express herself and sometimes she would yell and scream or flail her arms at me. There were fights, but there also was laughter, and there were tears from me for the mom I once knew, who no longer existed.

My husband and I had been planning to travel since before Mom had come to stay, and we decided that if we could make it work, we would still go. I looked for a temporary place for Mom, and I also asked my brother if he might be willing to take her for the three weeks we would be gone. Although I found a place for Mom, my brother said he would take her. I was surprised, but pleased.

Weeks after we returned, my brother and I got into a very heated argument over Mom. I was really angry and told my brother how poorly I thought he had handled some matters. Several days later, I received a letter from my brother saying I was no longer welcome in his house and that he and his family never wanted to see me again.

Mom stayed with me another year, until our paid caregiver wanted to move on. This time, *I* decided on my own that it was time for Mom to move into a nursing home. I felt she would do better in a smaller facility and there happened to be a fairly new one just a few blocks away. A visit there convinced me it would suit Mom and it was close enough so that I could stop by often.

Mom still had some sensibilities about her, so having to tell her that I couldn't take care of her anymore was really hard. She said, "OK, I'm going to do this, I'm going to try."

Physically moving her in, seeing her there, and then having to leave her, was difficult. Although people were going to look after her, I just knew this was the beginning of the end.

She was in the facility's Alzheimer's unit. She also was back in adult diapers. I hated that. She was dressing herself, so I would find her in all forms and strange combinations of dress. Sometimes she wouldn't put in her false teeth. I was told she helped the staff make the beds in the morning, which made sense to me because she always had to be doing something. Whenever I stopped by, she would break into a big smile and jump to her feet to come see me.

Mom had been in the facility for three months when she caught a cold, but this time, it developed into pneumonia. In the hospital, the pneumonia worsened significantly, and after about five days, I had her transferred to the hospice unit. I was in the hall introducing myself to the hospice nurses when Mom recognized my voice and called out that she wanted me in her room with her. She lay in bed surrounded by pillows. She was getting sleepy, so I told her I loved her and she said she loved me, too. Those were her last words, although she lived a few more days. On what was to be her last day, I watched as she kept reaching out her arms as if to say hello to long-lost loved ones. It seemed like she was being welcomed back to her family. I, on the other hand, was so very sad.

That my mom still knew me, even at the very end, was a wonderful gift that I treasure. But it was probably three or four years earlier when I recognized that the mom I knew was gone, and had said my goodbyes. You think you have already gone through the grief, but then, when they die and their physical presence is gone, you don't expect that to be as hard to say goodbye again. It was a few months before I actually laughed. We were visiting friends out of town and there was just so much joy and laughter that, all of a sudden, I was laughing and being joyous, too. I think at that moment, I realized how long it had been since I laughed; I mentioned it at the time to my husband, and he agreed.

Despite the many challenges and the losses—Mom's independence, our talks, and the relationship with my brother—I found my caregiving experience to be very rewarding. But I think there are some important lessons. First, not everyone is cut out for the role of caregiver, and that's okay. But it is so important for families to communicate.

In the beginning, my brother and I were working together, making decisions, talking. I've not spoken with him in about 12 years, since he declared me out of his life. Perhaps my brother and I should have had more discussions about the demands of caring for Mom. I know things would have turned out much differently between us. It actually is ironic because we saw my father and his sister become estranged after going through almost the same thing. My father was taking care of my grandma until one day his sister swooped in from out of town and took her away, and that was that. At the time, my brother and I said that this sort of thing would never happen to us.

The whole experience of caring for my mom has helped me grow, made me stronger in some ways, and helped me to understand some things. When issues arise, you have to be open to discussion; otherwise there can be misunderstandings, hurt feelings, and things can go wrong. Neither my brother nor I did a very good job communicating.

I'm glad that Mom was able to pass peacefully in her sleep. Sometimes death is especially painful and difficult, even when it doesn't have to be. I suppose the same can be said for caregiving.

Cris Abrams is a career businesswoman who has worked in industrial glass sales and financial services. She is currently employed in a company specializing in data aggregation for the real estate industry. She is a graduate of Katherine Gibbs School. Her mother, Margaret, was featured in HFA's program Living with Grief®: Alzheimer's Disease *in 2000.*

CHAPTER 7

Grief: A Companion on an Uncertain Journey

Kenneth J. Doka

Grief, the constant yet hidden companion of Alzheimer's disease and related dementias, can first arise with the realization that recent symptoms are *not* a normal part of aging and that something is wrong, or in the physician's office when a diagnosis is confirmed. Grief certainly will be experienced by family members as well, continuing as they view the slow deterioration in memory and the being of the person they love gradually slip away. The grief will increase as family members see a stranger emerge; a stranger who needs unceasing care, yet cannot recognize the caregiver. And grief will continue after the death, complicated by feelings that emerged over years, if not a decade, of caregiving. These feelings emanate from the family caregivers's own sense of losing someone they love who is still alive, guilt about decisions, and, perhaps, troubling feelings of relief and emancipation at the death. The grief may even be shared by professional caregivers who, in moments of intimate care, bonded with the individual with late-stage dementia as family members were already grieving the loss of the person they once knew.

This chapter considers issues of grief that arise in dementia. It begins by exploring ways that individuals with dementia grieve the reality of the advancing illness as well as how they grieve other losses encountered during their journey with dementia. The chapter then considers the grief of family members. The final section addresses clinical implications, noting ways that clinicians can assist grieving individuals, whether the person with dementia, a family caregiver, or a healthcare professional.

GRIEF AND THE PERSON WITH DEMENTIA

Anticipatory mourning in the course of dementia

Therese Rando (1986, 2000) reminds us that the term *anticipatory grief,* or as she prefers, *anticipatory mourning,* is paradoxically misunderstood yet useful. The misunderstanding comes when the term is seen simply as a reaction to an anticipated or future loss, where the concept of anticipatory mourning is limited to describing only how an individual reacts to the foreknowledge of an impending loss.

To Rando (2000), the term *anticipatory mourning* is useful when broadly referring to the reaction and response to all losses encountered in the past, present, or future of a life-threatening illness. These losses, and the grief reactions they evoke, are part of the daily experience of both those living with the disease as well as their family and caregiver.

These losses can be profound. First, there is the very real loss of the past; as one ceases to remember, links to the past are severed. One individual with dementia poignantly expressed this type of loss to his physician by crying out, "I used to remember!" as he struggled to recount an incident from childhood.

The deterioration of memory also affects the present. Memory links a person to another, allowing the ability to recall shared relationships and histories. Those with dementia eventually can no longer remember individuals around them, or are unable to recall or express relationships. For example, one woman with Alzheimer's disease had long been close with her daughter-in-law. Yet, as the disease progressed, she could only express the relationship as "the woman who married my son." This term caused a great deal of grief for the younger woman, as it seemingly invalidated what had been a long, positive relationship.

As memory lapses, other losses follow. One may no longer be able to function effectively in other roles; work and cherished activities may have to be relinquished. Couples frequently have to renegotiate their roles as progressive memory losses unfold (Robinson, Clare, & Evans, 2005). In addition, other relationships will change. The person with dementia and the family will need to decide how and to whom they will disclose the diagnosis. Some families begin to withdraw or isolate themselves from others (Robinson, Clare, & Evans, 2005). In the early stages of dementia, both the person with dementia and the family may experience these losses, but as the disease progresses, individuals with dementia often lose the ability to recognize loss and grief. The sense of specific loss and cognitive deterioration may be replaced by a vague feeling that something is wrong. This generalized sense may manifest in behaviors that evidence inner pain, such as agitation; as cognition declines, feelings and states of emotional stress remain (Rando, 1993).

Eventually, the individual with dementia may experience *psychological death* or the loss of individual consciousness. The person ceases to be aware of self. "Not only does he not know who he is—he does not know *that* he is" (Kalish, 1966, p. 247). Of course, others can only infer this state.

Experiencing grief

Even as individuals struggle with dementia, they may experience additional significant losses apart from the illness. Loved ones, such as spouses or siblings, may become ill, be hospitalized or institutionalized, or die.

The question is whether or not to inform the individual with dementia that a loss has occurred. We sometimes think that such information is an inherent right in relationships. Yet, to a person with dementia, this information may simply add pain or confusion. Individual cognitive functioning and social support need to be taken into account. Will the individual with dementia know that others are sad and grieving? Will the individual with dementia notice the absence of the person? When the loss is due to death, it may be better to spare the individual with dementia any additional grief if the deceased was not part of his or her daily life.

If the individual with dementia is to be informed of the loss, it should occur when the individual is rested and functioning well; generally, in the morning or after a good sleep. The news should be shared by a familiar, supportive person who will remain for whatever time is needed so the individual with dementia can process the information as much as capable without feeling abandoned.

Persons with dementia may be unable to retain the information that an individual has died. They may ask repeatedly what has occurred to that person and seemingly mourn the loss, only to reiterate the question later. In such cases, caregivers should acknowledge their own frustration and be reassured that such behaviors are normal in the disease and not indications of an inadequacy of explanations. One technique that can be useful is to return to a picture or memory each time the person with dementia questions the loss or expresses a sense of grief. Speaking of the person who has died in the past tense may also be helpful.

Unfortunately, there is little research that considers how an individual with dementia copes with loss. Persons with dementia may confuse the present loss with earlier losses. Herrmann and Grek (1988) documented two cases where bereaved spouses with dementia retained a delusional belief that a parent, rather than a spouse, had died. Rando (1993) emphasizes that the loss of cognition should not be compared with the absence of emotion. Grief in dementia may be evident in changes in behaviors as well as unusual or increased manifestations or even agitation or restlessness.

Expression of grief by an individual with dementia can be affected by a variety of factors, including the extent of disease and loss of awareness, certainty and immediacy of the lost relationship, and the ability to communicate the loss. It is critical to be sensitive to the loss; it has even been hypothesized that significant losses, as well as the inherent changes that occur as a secondary effect of loss, may exacerbate the dementia (Rando, 1993; Kastenbaum, 1969).

In dealing with losses experienced by persons with dementia, consider assuming an experimental ethos, constantly assessing what works best with a given individual at a particular time. Ritual and reminiscing about the person who died may be helpful; Lewis and Trzinski (2006) suggest two techniques that might facilitate processing. In *spaced retrieval*, new information is shared and then asked to be recalled over increasing intervals. In *group buddies*, an application of play therapy, the individual is given a stuffed animal to bring to a support group to "watch and learn." Clients then process information with their "buddies" following the group meetings. While both techniques may be helpful, ongoing assessment is essential to see if or how well they assist each person responding to loss.

Given the individuality of persons with dementia and varying cognitive functioning, there is no single approach that is universally applicable. For one person with dementia, keeping a photograph of the deceased to refer to whenever he or she asks about the individual can serve as a gentle reminder of the loss. For another person with dementia, removing the photograph may prevent repetitive questions and ongoing distress.

GRIEF AND FAMILY CAREGIVERS

During the illness

The concept of anticipatory mourning encompasses families of individuals with dementia as well. The losses the family experiences, and the grief engendered by these losses, will become more profound as the individual with dementia deteriorates (Ponder & Pomeroy, 1996; Meuser & Marwit, 2001). Families may perceive this as an *ambiguous loss*; the person is still alive but now changed (Boss, 2010). Here, families experience a deep sense of *psychosocial loss*; the persona of the person, or the psychological essence of individual personality, is perceived as lost although the person remains physically alive. The sense of individual identity has so changed that family members experience the death of the person who once was (Doka & Aber, 2002). Spouses may become *cryptowidows*, married in name but not in fact, and grieve losses associated with that role, such as intimacy, companionship, and sexuality (Doka & Aber, 2002; Teri & Reifler, 1986).

The very experience of caregiving may complicate grief. As caregivers, individuals may experience secondary losses such as social and recreational roles, work roles, and relationships with others. The increased demands of caring for someone with a progressive illness, and the experience of psychosocial loss and possibly secondary losses, may generate an unceasing state of grief, sometimes identified as chronic sorrow (Roos, 2002; Mayer, 2001; Burke, Hainsworth, Eakes & Lindgren, 1992; Loos & Bowd, 1997) and reactive depression (Walker & Pomeroy, 1996).

For many family caregivers, the decision to place their loved one with dementia in a facility can complicate grieving. Reactions to the loss generated by institutionalization can include responses such as relief, guilt, and failure. Professional caregivers can assist early in the process by encouraging families to "draw a line in the sand" by defining in advance when taking care of the person at home will become too difficult. Such a question plants a seed that future institutionalization may be unavoidable as their loved one's condition continues to deteriorate. Most families generally go beyond what they initially believed was possible; this "delayed" institutionalization is seen as a success rather than failure. Professional caregivers can also help families redefine their caregiving role *after* institutionalization; they are still caregivers, but their role changes from provider of direct care to that of advocate. There may be other decisions, too, that will generate guilt and complicate grief. Moreover, the long-term effects of caregiving can diminish coping abilities, and the constant demands of care may limit social support (Bodnar & Kiecolt-Glaser, 1994).

Dementia also affects caregiver grief in another way. As individuals with dementia deteriorate, their ability to monitor and regulate their behavior diminishes. Some exhibit a range of unusual behaviors such as using foul language or indecent and inappropriate actions. They may relive earlier traumas. For example, some Holocaust survivors experiencing the symptoms of Alzheimer's disease began to hoard food, experience troubling flashbacks, or have a heightened sense of anxiety (McCann, 2003). People with dementia may express attitudes that were once self-censored, such as engaging in racial or personal diatribes. These behaviors can humiliate, embarrass, and isolate caregivers, increasing ambivalence and discomfort that subsequently complicates grief.

Grief at the time of death

When the person with dementia dies, grief changes focus. Some people experience a *liberating loss* (Jones & Martinson, 1992; Elison & McGonigle, 2003), characterized by feelings of relief and emancipation that caregiving responsibilities and suffering by both the patient and family have ended.

Some may actually grieve the loss of the caregiving role, and feel a lack of focus and meaninglessness in their activities. For some, these feelings are accompanied by guilt and sadness. Survivors may reminisce about the caregiving experience, reflecting on times that they might have shown more patience or empathy. They might believe that there was more that they could have done, or regret hurtful things that were said. Such memories, while common and understandable, are related to greater depression, stress, and social isolation (Bodnar & Kiecolt-Glaser, 1994).

This grief may not only be manifested in affect, but in cognition, behavior, and spirituality. It may be experienced physically; health consequences do not end with the change in the caregiving role. In fact, increased medical symptoms in caregivers are associated with transitions from this role, such as nursing home placement or death of the person with Alzheimer's disease (Grant, Adler, Patterson, Dimsdale, Ziegler, & Irwin, 2002).

Others may disenfranchise the grief that caregivers and people with dementia experience. *Disenfranchised grief* refers to losses that are not appreciated by others. The individual has no perceived "right" to mourn; the loss is not openly acknowledged or socially sanctioned and publicly shared. Others simply do not understand why this loss is mourned and may fail to validate and support grief (Doka, 1989, 2002).

Grief resulting from the death of a person with dementia can be disenfranchised for a number of reasons. Often, the person with Alzheimer's disease or another dementia is devalued; he or she is seen as old, confused, or burdensome. Death may be seen as a release for both the caregiver and the person who died, or survivors may be expected to have grieved already in the course of the illness. Even customary statements of sympathy and support may be tinged with ambivalent sentiments like, "This is a blessing," or "It must be a great relief," without understanding the impact of the loss and the depth of survivors' grief. A wide range of factors, including the circumstances surrounding the loss, past coping capacities and grieving styles, as well as other social and psychological variables, will affect the nature and extent of grief (Worden, 2009; Rando, 1993; Martin & Doka, 2000). Ethnicity and culture certainly play a role. For example, Owen, Goode, and Haley (2001) found that African-American caregivers, when compared to white caregivers, were more likely to experience higher levels of grief.

Other research has noted that manifestations of grief were different between those whose partner with dementia was maintained at home compared to those who placed their partner in a nursing home. Those who provided care in the home reported exhaustion, stress, anxiety, and anger; partners of individuals placed in nursing homes indicated higher levels of guilt and sadness (Rudd, Viney, & Presten, 1999; Collins, Liken, King, & Kokinakis, 1993).

While many influences can mediate the experience of grief, one fact remains: grief is a constant companion to Alzheimer's disease and dementia up to and following death. The goal of support is to acknowledge and validate the loss—to enfranchise grief.

Grief and professional caregivers

Grief is not based solely on familial ties; grief is based on attachment. It is not unusual for professional caregivers to become attached to their patients, and thus experience grief. This grief can be particularly intense among caregivers likely to be more involved in the daily care of the patient, such as home health aides or nursing assistants.

This reality can create a paradoxical situation. As family members grieve the loss of the individual they once knew, aides or other professional caregivers become attached to the person with dementia they see today. This can cause certain ethical quandaries. In one situation, a well-known and respected attorney and judge was institutionalized in the final stage of dementia. Her family deeply grieved the loss of a brilliant woman and devoted mother. Yet, as her dementia progressed, she thought every staff member in the facility was family and treated them as such, kissing and thanking them for every kindness. The staff grew to love her. Her advance directives were written with great clarity, indicating her wish not to be treated for certain conditions as she entered the end-stage of Alzheimer's disease, so when she developed pneumonia, the ethics committee of the facility and her family agreed that the advance directives should be honored, but the staff was demoralized by her death (Doka, 1994).

Enfranchising grief

In validating grief, it is critical to revisit two points: grief is experienced in varying ways by the person with dementia, the family and professional caregivers; grief is encountered throughout the illness as well as after the death. Thus, assistance and support should be offered to all involved both during the illness and following death.

Two considerations are essential in offering support to persons with dementia: validation and control. When an individual is diagnosed with dementia, his or her anxiety, anger, or other manifestations of grief may be discounted and denied. Often, this is done to protect the person by offering glib reassurance that everything is fine, even when the individual with dementia is aware and fearful of manifestations of the disease.

This response is unhelpful. Persons in the early stages of dementia have very clear awareness of the symptoms of decline; even later in the illness, individuals may have vague feelings of loss of certain capabilities. Empathetic listening, expressions of support, reassuring remembrance that reaffirms relationships, and, when appropriate, physical touch, can validate and show support.

Another way to respect an individual with dementia is by helping him or her retain a sense of control. An individual feeling abilities slip away may be determined to maintain as much control of the environment as possible. In the early stages of dementia, there may be expressions of anticipatory bereavement (Gerber, 1974) or actions clearly indicating the need to plan for impending losses. The individual may want to finish business by contacting associates, give instructions to family, and review or create advance directives. All of this should be supported. However, not every person chooses to confront feelings or plan for the future, which also is a way to cope.

Provide education about the underlying condition

There are many strategies to assist family members as they cope with the inevitable losses associated with dementia (Doka & Aber, 2002). It is important to assess each person's perception of the affected individual's underlying condition because often, the family's understanding of that condition is faulty. Through this exploration, counselors can determine whether each family member's perspective of the diagnosis and prognosis sustains false hopes or unrealistic beliefs (e.g., that the person can control behavior or will get better).

Exploring each family member's beliefs gives counselors the opportunity to provide education at each person's level. Counselors should be prepared to suggest resources, such as organizations, self-help groups, and particularly, books by people who have experienced similar loss. Such education not only provides realistic information about the nature and course of the disease, it can also enhance feelings of coping and control by allowing family members a sense of meaningful activity and by providing them with opportunities to anticipate and plan contingencies.

Offer support for coping with the emotional issues related to the loss

Family members often feel constrained in recognizing and expressing their emotions. Because the person with dementia may live in the same community or the same home, family members may lack opportunity to express negative emotions, or face social sanctions from friends and relatives who consider such expressions disloyal or unfeeling.

The experience of caregiving can engender strong emotions. Caregivers may feel angry or resentful toward the person with dementia, or may be hurt by a perceived lack of support from others. They may feel guilt from their ambivalence about caregiving or any feelings of relief and emancipation after the person with dementia has died. Counselors can help by creating a nonjudgmental atmosphere where individuals can express and explore these complicated emotions. In addition to reassurance that such feelings are normal, counselors can offer strategies such as journal writing, participation in ritual, or sharing such feelings with an empty chair representing the person who has died. These strategies can help grievers cope with a wide range of feelings.

Help family members respond to change

Throughout the progression of dementia, people experience many changes as well as losses in their daily lives. Dealing with the constant demands of the illness often means a change in the ability to participate in previously enjoyed activities; loss of pleasurable companionship and loss of contact with friends or relatives; the need to take on new and challenging responsibilities; changes in expectations for the future; and the reality of unmet psychological, social, sexual, and financial needs.

After the death, family caregivers can experience additional losses, including the meaningful role as caregiver. These changes can occur so quickly that persons neither realize just how profoundly their own lives have been altered nor have the time to develop effective coping strategies. The simple question, "In what ways has your life changed?" can release a flood of responses. Counselors can assist individuals in determining which of these secondary losses are most significant; what opportunities exist to regain, to whatever extent, some of what has been lost; and help explore responses and strategies for dealing with such losses.

Counselors can also discuss the nature of the family caregiver's support systems. Family members should be encouraged to explore how their support system can provide strategies for respite and resumption of missed activity; how to better utilize the supports they have in place, which may allow further discussion of coping styles and problem-solving abilities; and "surprises" in the support system, including both unexpected sources of support as well as support that did not come through as anticipated. This last issue is particularly significant as it provides further opportunity for the counselor to discuss emotional responses such as anger and resentment, as well as focus on personal problem-solving skills and coping strategies.

Upon assessment, individuals may recognize that they did not adequately communicate their needs or feelings to others in their support system, or that they relied on others in inappropriate ways. In one case, a woman angered by her daughter's seeming inability to listen to complaints about the caregiving demands resulting from her husband's dementia realized upon reflection that her daughter's strengths were always in "active doing" rather than "passive listening." Once the woman recognized this reality, she was able to modify her expectations and found that her daughter was extremely supportive when asked to help with active tasks, such as providing rides for her father or running errands.

Counselors also assist families by finding additional sources of support, such as self-help groups, day care and respite programs, and, if necessary, institutional care. These additional supports can help reduce stress and allow family members to take direct actions that may diminish guilt and reaffirm control. Support groups have been particularly successful for caregivers as well as for persons who are newly-diagnosed with Alzheimer's disease (Wasow & Coons, 1987; Simank & Strickland, 1986; Yale, 1989). The groups decrease isolation, facilitate grief, and enable exchange of information and resources. But counselors must do more than simply identify needs and sources of support; in some cases, counselors need to explore resistance and ambivalence toward such support. As Quayhagen and Quayhagen (1988) note, some caregivers experience considerable guilt over leaving the care of the person to others, and accepting help from formal agencies may no longer allow the defense of denial.

Counselors can explore role problems, dilemmas, and ambiguities within families. One of the most significant problems of dementia, especially for spouses, is that it creates considerable role strain and generates additional burden. For example, the spouse may be legally married though effectively widowed because the companionship and sexuality that were part of the prior relationship no longer exist. In these situations, it often is helpful for the spouse to explore the tensions, ambiguities, burdens, and difficulties that accompany this state of cryptowidowhood.

Counselors also can encourage such caregivers to explore all possible options. Even if an option is precluded for moral or practical reasons, its very consideration reaffirms a sense of control and reduces the feeling that the future is totally constrained. In one case, a woman whose husband was institutionalized with Alzheimer's disease became involved in a relationship with another man, but decided she would neither divorce her spouse nor live with her new love. However, acknowledging both options allowed her to affirm that she has some control over events and that decisions she makes now are not necessarily final.

Counselors can be helpful by discussing ways an individual generally copes with change and how the individual is coping with it now; by helping individuals assess which strategies are effective and reaffirming and reinforcing such skills; by providing opportunities to assess, improve or develop better strategies; and by looking at ways the caregiver deals with stress, teaching effective stress-reduction techniques if needed. Counselors also can help caregivers to consider the impact of decisions made around caregiving. For example, an individual's decision to quit work to take care of a spouse with dementia may remove him or her from a support system, eliminate necessary respite, and create financial problems. Counselors should assist individuals periodically in assessing caregiving plans and roles, and in reviewing alternatives. Finally, counselors can legitimize the needs of family members and help them to recognize and balance their own needs with the demands of caregiving.

Help families plan realistically for the future

The nature of dementia often encourages an attitude of living "one day at a time." In many ways, such a perspective is functional; with a progressive disease like dementia, the future can be dismal. Nevertheless, it is important for families to plan, as that allows a sense of control and provides opportunity to rehearse problem-solving skills, anticipate issues, and conduct necessary research and information-gathering. Counselors facilitate the family's planning process when assisting family members through change, as noted earlier; by reaffirming confidence in the individual's abilities, coping skills, and realistic hopes; and by allowing family members to explore the effects of change on their own sense of self, sense of others, and their beliefs.

Alzheimer's disease and dementia can profoundly alter views of self or of others, and fundamental beliefs about faith and meaning. Caregivers may be fearful of their own future; they may question their feelings and beliefs about other family members, perhaps experiencing disappointment in the reaction or support of others.

As caregivers cope with changes wrought by the illness, they may have troubling experiences with the person who has dementia, such as uncovering unusual behaviors or attitudes. In one case, a woman was clearly discomforted by her mother's negative reactions to persons of a different race. Prior to developing dementia, her mother had been a strong supporter of the civil rights movement and had never expressed such an attitude. Caregivers in similar instances need space and opportunity to confront their emotions and reconstruct meaning. A good beginning would be asking questions such as, "How does this affect your beliefs about yourself and your family or your beliefs about the world?" Assignments in which clients seek out information or enter into discussion with others, including members of their own faith community, can facilitate this process. Tasks such as assembling videos or photo albums can reconnect individuals to earlier, more positive memories.

In addition to family members, it also is important to offer support to professional caregivers. Since many dementias progress over a long period of time, it is not unusual for nursing home aides, home companions, and home health aides to develop strong relationships with family members as well as with the person with dementia. When that person dies, the aide not only ends a relationship with the individual, but often with the family as well. Health aides lose a position and income and may need to develop another relationship almost immediately. In cases of advanced dementia when healthcare decisions have been made, the aide's perspective often is not expressed and would, in some circumstances, be unwelcome. Yet, professional caregivers mourn, too. Their grief needs to be acknowledged and supported by the agencies that employ them. Tangible ways to support such staff include debriefings following an assignment, sharing thank-you notes from the family, and personnel policies that encourage participation in memorials, funerals, or other rituals.

Grief is a constant companion to individuals with dementia and their families. From the first realization that this diagnosis may be a possibility, to the death of the person with the disease, loss is integrally woven in to the experience. Grief impacts the person coping with the disease, even in the later stages of the illness. Grief is also present for the family caregivers and loved ones, who experience losses not only of the person they love, but losses of familiar roles and dreams for the future. Professional caregivers are also touched by grief and may not always have the support they need to integrate those reactions into their daily work.

But grief does not have to be the only companion. As family and friends, counselors, and supportive others travel together, the journey through grief continues, but is perhaps less lonely and not quite as frightening.

Editor's Note: This chapter draws material from Doka, K. J. (2004). Grief in Dementia. In K. J. Doka (Ed.), Living with grief: Alzheimer's disease (pp. 139-154). Washington, DC: Hospice Foundation of America.

Kenneth J. Doka, PhD, MDiv, *is a professor of gerontology at the Graduate School of The College of New Rochelle and senior consultant to Hospice Foundation of America. Dr. Doka serves as editor of HFA's* Living with Grief® *book series, its* Journeys *newsletter, and numerous other books and publications. Dr. Doka has served as a panelist on HFA's* Living with Grief® *video programs for 22 years. He is a past president of the Association for Death Education and Counseling (ADEC) and recently received their Special Contributions Award. He is a member and past chair of the International Work Group on Death, Dying and Bereavement. In 2006, Dr. Doka was grandfathered in as a mental health counselor under New York's first state licensure of counselors. Dr. Doka is an ordained Lutheran minister.*

REFERENCES

Bodnar, J. C., & Kiecolt-Glaser, J. K. (1994). Caregiver depression after bereavement: Chronic stress isn't over when it's over. *Psychology & Aging, 9,* 372-380.

Boss, P. (2010). The trauma and complicated grief of ambiguous loss. *Pastoral Psychology, 59,* 137-145.

Burke, M. L., Hainsworth, M. A., Eakes, G. G., & Lindgren, C. L. (1992). Current knowledge and research in chronic sorrow: A foundation for inquiry. *Death Studies, 16,* 231-245.

Collins, C., Liken, M., King, S. O., & Kokinakas, C. (1993). Loss and grief among family caregivers or relatives with dementia. *Qualitative Health Research 3,* 236-253.

Doka, K. J. (Ed.) (1989). *Disenfranchised grief: Recognizing hidden sorrow.* Lexington, MA: Lexington Books.

Doka, K. J. (1994). Caregiver distress: If it is so ethical, why does it feel so bad? *Critical Issues in Clinical Care Nursing, 5,* 346-7.

Doka, K. J. (Ed.). (2002). *Disenfranchised grief: New directions, challenges and strategies for practice.* Champaign, IL: Research Press.

Doka, K. J., & Aber, R. (2002). Psychological loss and grief. In K. J. Doka (Ed.), *Disenfranchised grief: New directions, challenges and strategies for practice.* Champaign, IL. : Research Press.

Elison, J., & McGonigle, C. (2003). *Liberating losses: When death brings relief.* Cambridge, MA: Perseus Publishing.

Gerber, I. (1976). Anticipating bereavement. In B. Schoenberg, A. Carr, A. Kurscher, D. Peretz, & I. Goldberg (Eds.) *Anticipatory grief.* New York, NY: Columbia University Press.

Grant, I., Adler, K., Patterson, T. L., Dimsdale, J. E., Ziegler, M. G., & Irwin, M. R. (2002). Health consequences & Alzheimer's caregiving transitions: Effects of placement and bereavement. *Psychosomatic Medicine, 64,* 477-486.

Herrmann, N., & Grek, A. (1988). Delusional double mourning: A complication of bereavement in dementia. *Canadian Journal of Psychiatry, 33,* 851-852.

Jones, P. S., & Martinson, I. (1992). The experience of bereavement in caregiving of family members with Alzheimer's disease. *IMAGE: Journal of Nursing Scholarship, 214,* 172-176.

Kalish, R. A. (1966). A continuum of subjectively perceived death. *The Gerontologist, 6,* 73-76.

Kastenbaum, R. (1969). Death and bereavement in later life. In A. Kutscher (Ed.), *Death and the elderly.* Springfield, IL: Thomas.

Lewis, M., & Trzinski, A. (2006). Counseling older adults with dementia who are dealing with death: Innovative interventions for practitioners. *Death Studies, 30,* 777-787.

Loos, C., & Bowd, A. (1997). Caregivers of persons with Alzheimer's disease: Some neglected implications of the experience of personal loss and grief. *Death Studies, 21,* 501-514.

Martin, T., & Doka, K. J. (2000). *Men don't cry, women do: Transcending gender stereotypes of grief.* Philadelphia, PA: Brunner/Mazel.

Mayer, M. (2001). Chronic sorrow in caregiving spouses of patients with Alzheimer's disease. *Journal of Aging and Identity, 6,* 49-60.

McCann, T. (2003). Holocaust survivors with Alzheimer's can relive old horrors. Retrieved from http://www.Sanlvisobispo.com/mrd/sanlvisobispo/news/nation/por690.btm

Meuser, T., & Marwit, S. (2001). A comprehensive, stage-sensitive model of grief in dementia caregiving. *The Gerontologist, 40,* 678-670.

Owen, J. E., Goode, K. T., & Haley, W. E. (2001). End-of-life care and reactions to death in African-American and White family caregivers of relatives with Alzheimer's disease. *Omega: Journal of Death and Dying, 43,* 348-361.

Quayhagan, M. P., & Quayhagan, M. (1988). Alzheimer's stress: Coping with the caregiver role. *The Gerontologist, 28,* 391-396.

Ponder, R. J., & Pomeroy, E. C. (1966). The grief of caregivers: How pervasive is it? *Journal of Gerontological Social Work, 27,* 3-21.

Rando, T. A. (1986). *Loss and anticipatory grief.* Lexington, MA: Lexington Books.

Rando, T. A. (1993). *The treatment of complicated mourning.* Champaign, IL: Research Press.

Rando, T. A. (2000). *Clinical dimensions of anticipatory mourning: Theory and practice in working with the dying, their loved ones and their caregivers.* Champaign, IL: Research Press.

Robinson, I., Clare, L., & Evans, K. (2005). Making sense of dementia and adjusting to loss: Psychological reactions to the diagnosis of dementia in couples. *Aging & Mental Health, 9,* 337-347.

Roos, S. (2002). *Chronic sorrow: A living loss.* New York, NY: Routledge.

Rudd, M. G., Viney, L. L, .& Presten, C. A. (1999). The grief expressed by spousal caregivers of dementia patients: The role of place of care of patient and gender of the patient. *International Journal of Aging & Human Development, 48,* 217-240.

Simank, M. H. & Strickland, K. J. (1986). Assisting families in coping with Alzheimer's disease and other related dementias with the establishment of a mutual support group. *The Journal of Gerontological Social Work, 9*(2), 49-58.

Teri, L. V. & Reifler, B. V. (1986). Sexual issues of patients with Alzheimer's disease. *Medical Aspects of Human Sexuality, 20*, 86-91.

Vennen, A., Shanks, M. F., Staff, M. F., & Sala, S. D. (2000). Nurturing syndrome: A form of pathological bereavement with delusions in Alzheimer's disease. N*europsychological, 38*, 213-224.

Walker, R. J., & Pomeroy, F. C. (1996). Depression or grief?: The experience of caregivers of people with dementia. *Health & Social Work, 21*, 247-254.

Wasow, M., & Coons, D. M (1987). Widows and widowers of Alzheimer's victims: Their survival after a spouse's deaths. *Journal of Independent Social Work, 2*, 21-32.

Worden, W. W. (2009). *Grief counseling and grief therapy* (4th Ed). New York, NY: Springer.

Yale, R. (1989). Support groups for newly diagnosed Alzheimer's clients. *Clinical Gerontologist, 18*, 86-89.

Index

R

S

T